101 Raw Food Recipes From Nomad Rose

Regain Your Health Through Real Nutrition

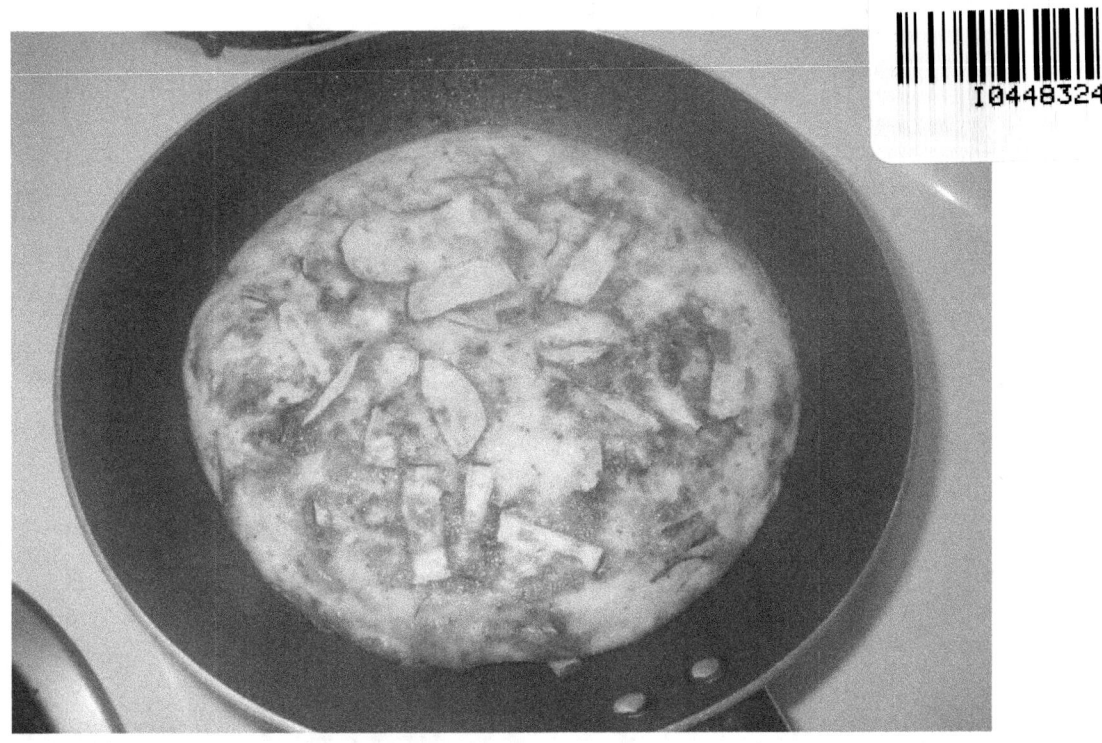

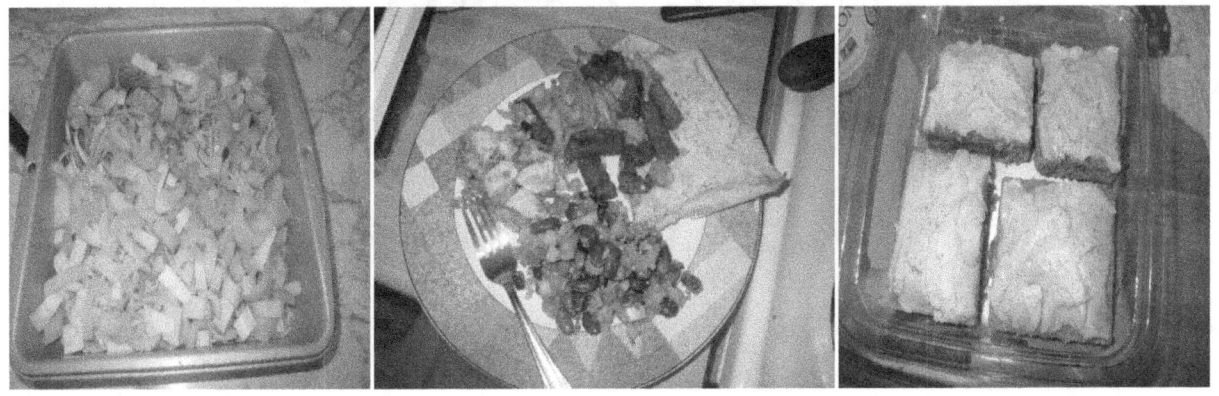

CHECK OUT HEALTH ARTICLES, WORKOUT TIPS AND MORE AT NOMADROSE.COM

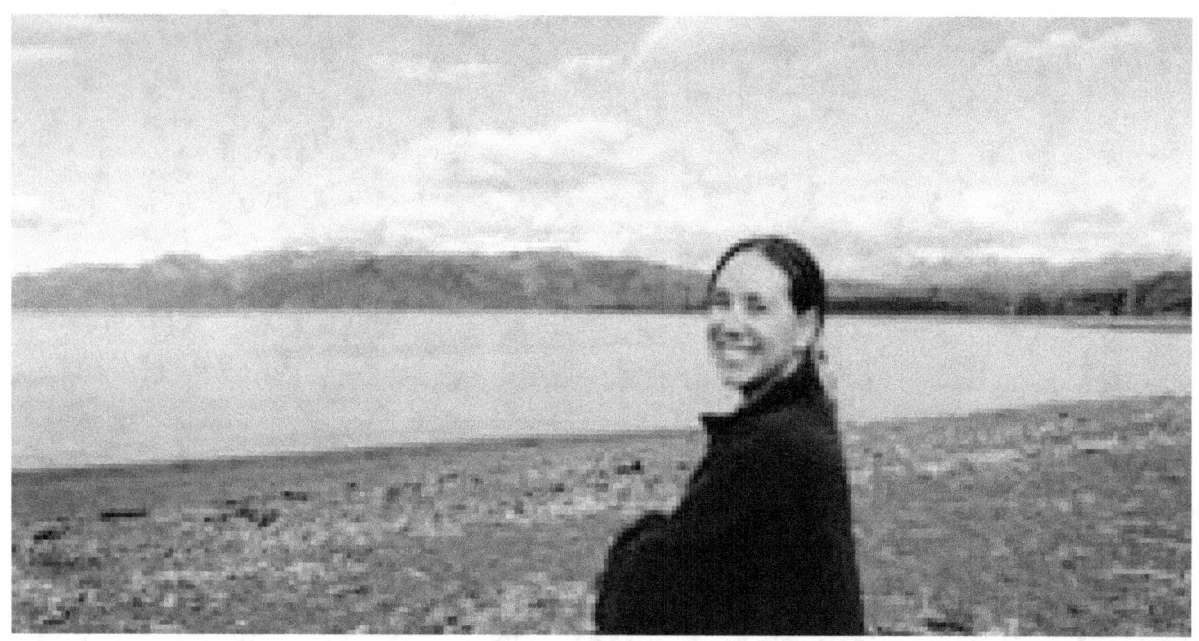

101 Raw Food Recipes From Nomad Rose

Regain Your Health Through Real Nutrition

Rose Short

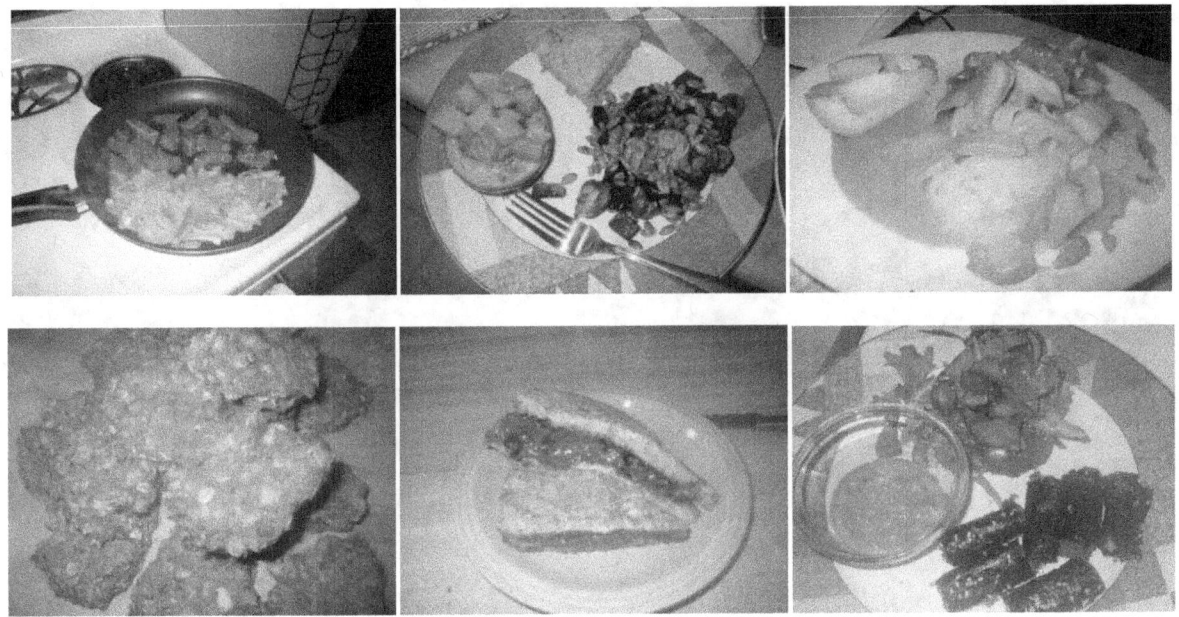

Rose's Live Real Advice

2016

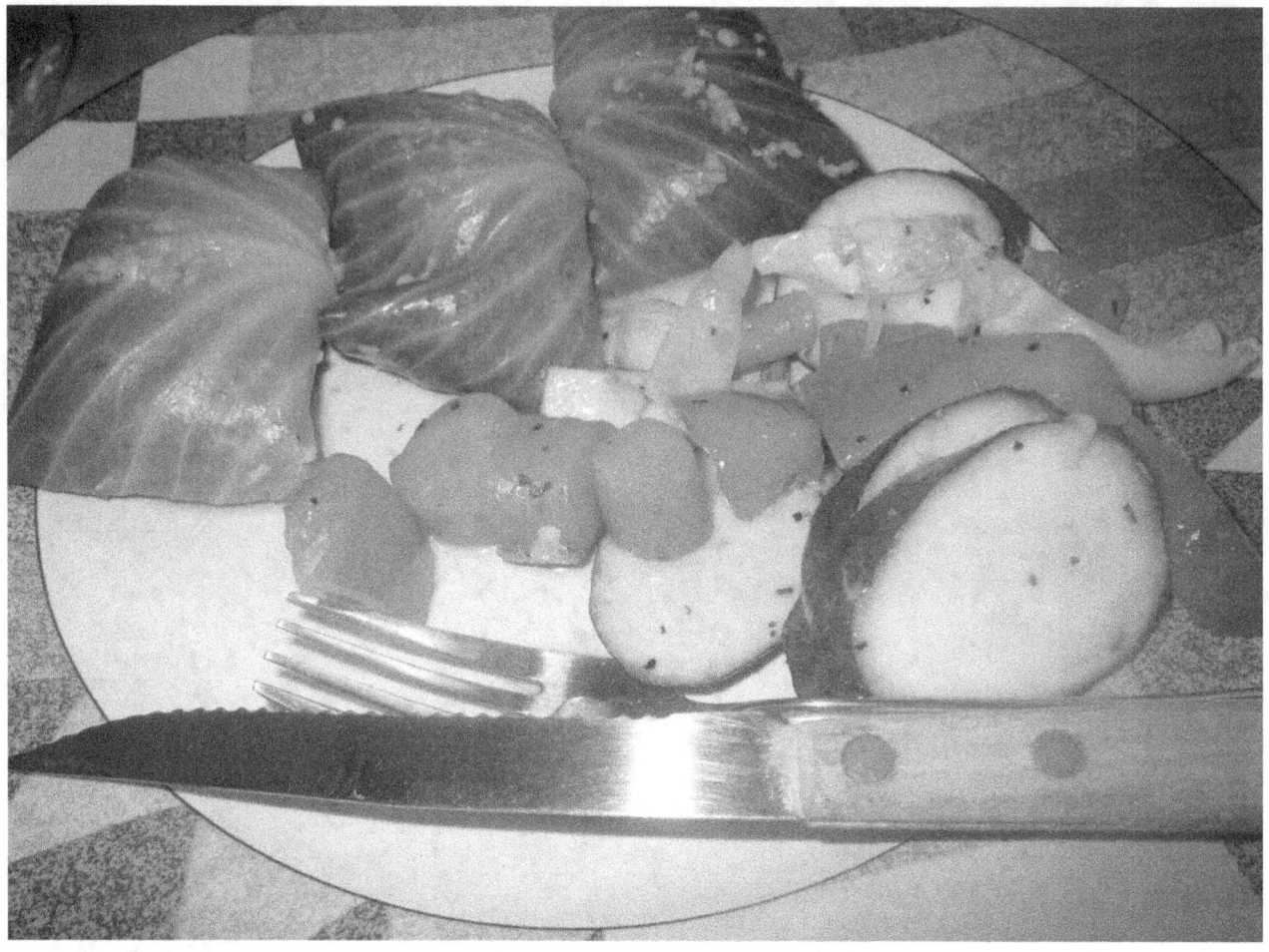

FIRST PRINTING: 2016

ISBN 978-1-365-07164-5

ROSE'S LIVE REAL ADVICE
64 HAZEL DR
RIVERTON , WYOMING 82501

WWW.NOMADROSE.COM

Contents

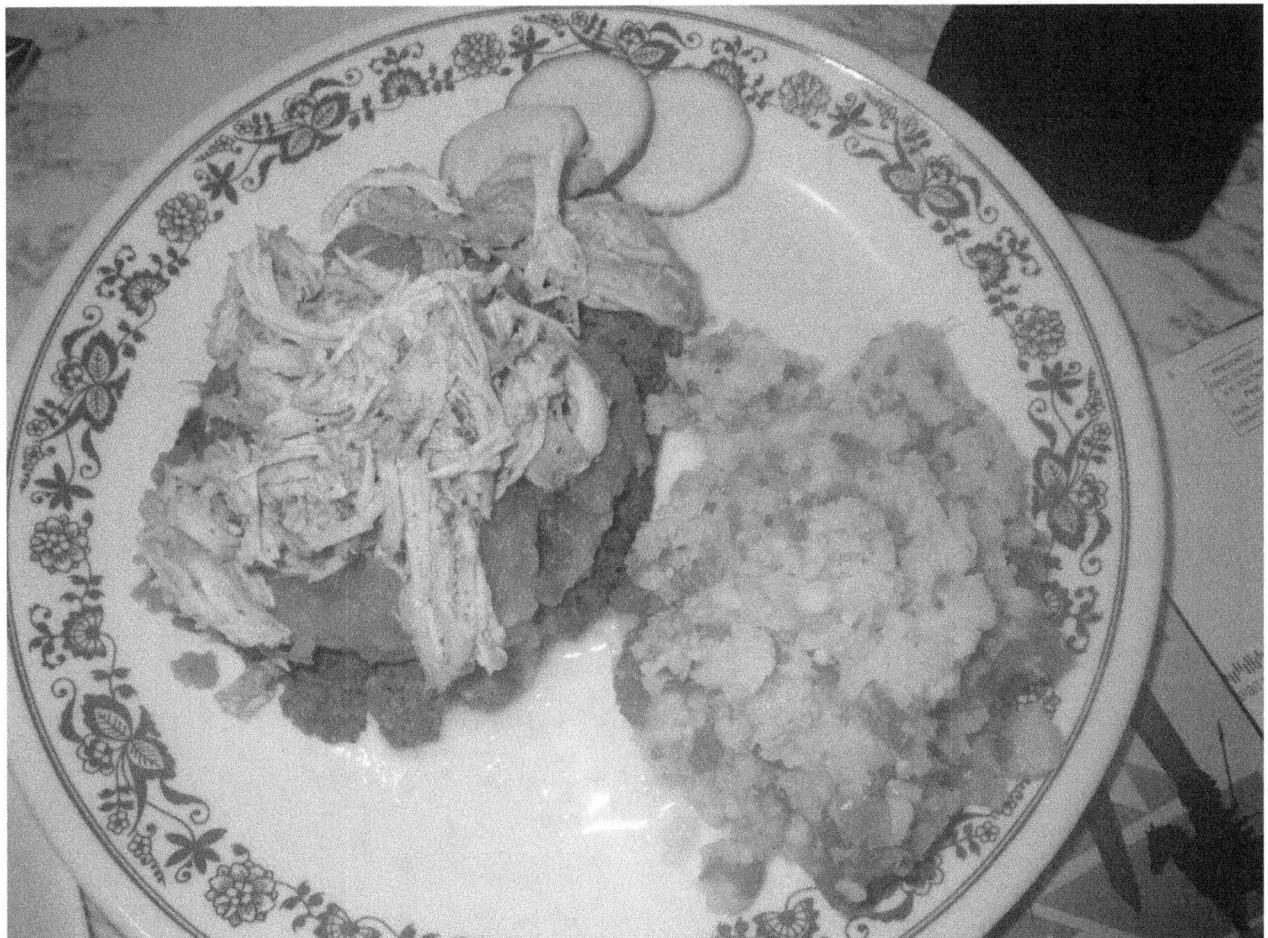

Welcome To My Whole Food Kitchen!!

This is my first book so I apologise in advance if it is a little strange; I am still getting used to explaining every move I make in the kitchen. I have included a broad range of foods that are easy to make, delicious, and healthy. I have included the best nutrition information available to me, and I believe it to be accurate. The nutrition will change as you sub ingredients of course but all ingredients are fairly easy to sub out, so don't be afraid to experiment.

I have broken the book into catagories of benefit rather than meal times because, honestly, I love breakfast for dinner. I don't believe people should place stipulations on healthy choices based on time of day; if you want a vegretable salad for breakfast, go for it!

There are links at nomadrose.com that will take you to the sites where some of my ingredients are available: Green drink powders, protein powders, etc.

I hope you enjoy!

Veggie Roasting Tips

Roasted Veggies: Good rule of thumb is 375 degrees F for 30-45 minutes, but here are some more specific roasting instructions.

Beetroot: Preheat oven to 400 degrees F. Rinse and cut off the tops, leaving an inch of stalk, and the bottoms. Place on a lined cookie sheet. Bake for 45 minutes. Check after 30 as you may need to turn them for even roasting. Use a fork to check for tenderness; if they are still raw they will have an earthy aftertaste rather than being sweet.

Squash: Preheat oven to 375 degrees F. Cut in half, scoop out the seeds, sprinkle with water, and place cut side down on a lined cookie sheet. Bake for 35-45 minutes; you don't want the skin to get too well done. When the skin is soft but not squishy, turn the squah over and bake an extra 5-15 minutes, being careful to not dehydrate.

Avocado: Preaheat oven to 425 degrees F. Cut open and remove the pit. If you are stuffing them, remove enough excess meat to make room for stuffing. Bake cooked side up for 15-25 minutes.

Liquid Vitamins

Acai Bowl

Acai Smoothie

Almond Butter Protein Bowl

Carrot Cake Chia Shake

Citrus Smoothie

Dragon Fruit Frozen Coconut Cream

Fruity Vitamin Smoothie

Ice Banana Coffee Mash

Pumpkin Pie Shake

Super Veggie Smoothie

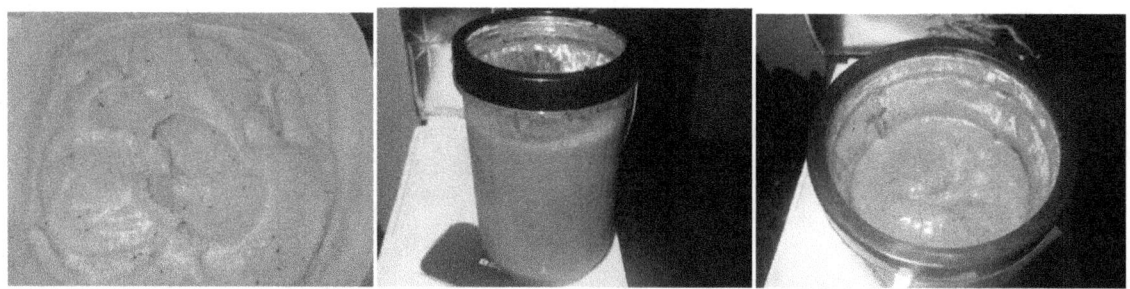

ACAI BOWL

Prep Time	5 Minutes
Cook /Chill Time	10 minutes for Bowl
Cook Temp (F)	NA
Servings	1
Storage	NA
Storage Duration	NA

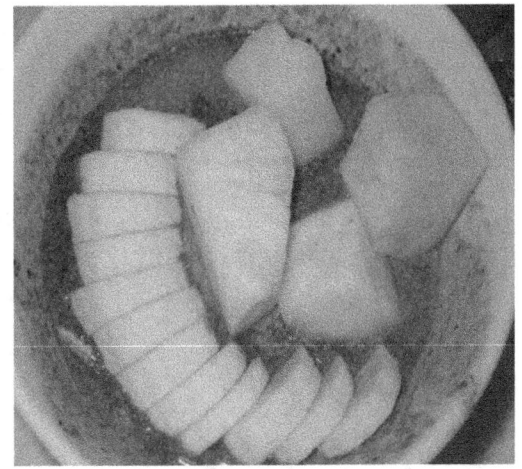

INGREDIENTS:

¼ cup fresh or frozen Pomegranate
¼ cup fresh of frozen Blueberries
¼-¾ cup Thai Lite Coconut Milk, chilled
1 Frozen Acai Smoothi Pack

INSTRUCTIONS:

Place a bowl in the freezer to help keep sorbet at frozen temperature. Combine all ingredients in a blender and blend smooth. Start with a low amount of milk and adjust as consistency will vary based on temperature of fruits. Pour into chilled bowl and enjoy.

VARIATIONS/SUGGESTIONS:

- Top with granola/honey/sliced fresh fruit/bee pollen/nuts
- Add protein powder if you use it

BASIC NUTRITION AND KEY VITAMINS/MINERALS PER SERVING							
Calories	Carbs (g)	Net Carbs (g)	Sugar (g)	Protein (g)	Fiber (g)	Fat (g)	Vitamins/Mineral
204	32	27	26	2	5	8	A, C, B's, Potassium

Acai Smoothie

Prep Time	5 Minutes
Cook /Chill Time	NA
Cook Temp (F)	NA
Servings	1
Storage	Refrigerate
Storage Duration	1 Day

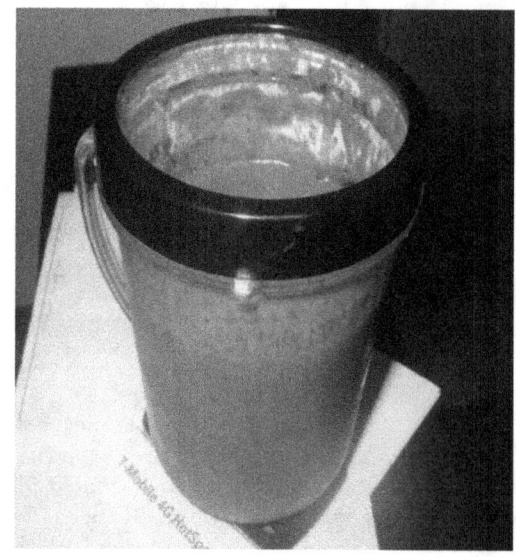

INGREDIENTS:

1 Acai Smoothie Pack
1 tsp Flax
1 tsp Chia Seed
¼ cup Pomegranate
1 cup Unsweetened Almond Milk
1 Tbsp Unsweetened Shredded Coconut

INSTRUCTIONS:

Place all ingredients into a blender and blend until smooth.

VARIATIONS/SUGGESTIONS:

- Add any other fruits you like
- Add protein powder for a great after workout shake

BASIC NUTRITION AND KEY VITAMINS/MINERALS PER SERVING							
Calories	Carbs (g)	Net Carbs (g)	Sugar (g)	Protein (g)	Fiber (g)	Fat (g)	Vitamins/Mineral
295	36	25	23	6	11	15	C, E, Bs, Copper

ALMOND BUTTER PROTEIN BOWL

Prep Time	5 Minutes
Cook /Chill Time	NA
Cook Temp (F)	NA
Servings	1
Storage	Refrigerate
Storage Duration	1 Day

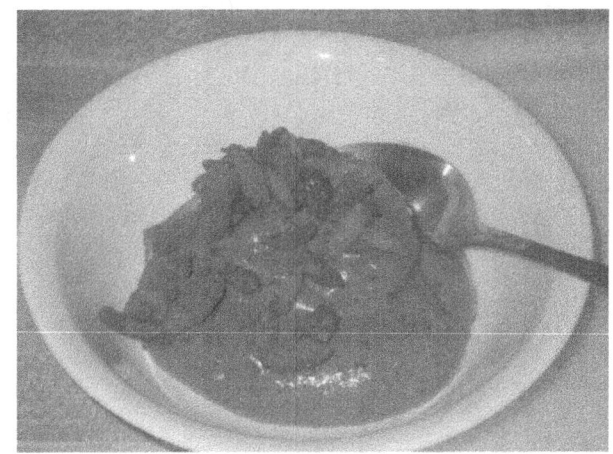

INGREDIENTS:

1 Scoop Yoli Yes Shake Vanilla or Chocolate
2 Tbsp Almond Butter
½ cup Unsweetened Almond Milk
2 tsp Flax
2 Tsp Chia Seed
1 Banana

INSTRUCTIONS:

Combine all ingredients in a blender and blend to thick, smooth consistancy.

VARIATIONS/SUGGESTIONS:

- Top with granola/seeds/fruit
- Sub dates or figs if you are not a fan of bananas
- Add raw honey for extra sweetness if desired

BASIC NUTRITION AND KEY VITAMINS/MINERALS PER SERVING							
Calories	Carbs (g)	Net Carbs (g)	Sugar (g)	Protein (g)	Fiber (g)	Fat (g)	Vitamins/Mineral
473	49	34	22	22	15	26	B2, E, D, Iron

CARROT CAKE CHIA SHAKE

Prep Time	5 Minutes
Cook /Chill Time	NA
Cook Temp (F)	NA
Servings	1
Storage	Refrigerate
Storage Duration	1 Day

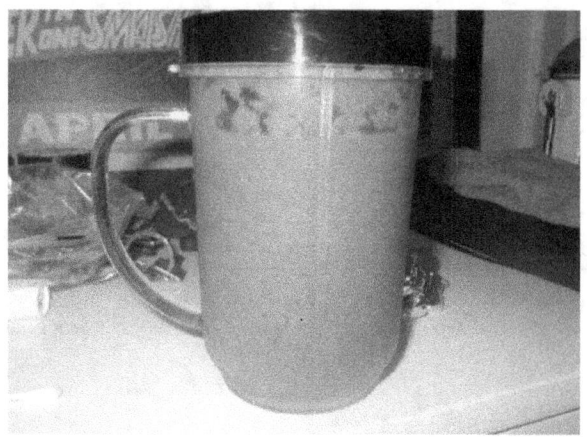

INGREDIENTS:

 2 medium peeled and diced carrots
 1 cup Unsweetened Almond Milk
 1 tsp Chia Seed
 1 tsp Flax
 1 tsp ground Cloves
 1 tsp cinnamon
 1 tsp ground Ginger
 1 tsp Nutmeg

INSTRUCTIONS:

Blend all ingredients in a blender or food processor that can handle raw carrots. If you don't have one, steam or roast the carrots ahead of time to make it easier to blend.

VARIATIONS/SUGGESTIONS:

- Use ¼ cup of carrot juice if you have some
- Adjust spices to fit your taste
- Add protein powder if you like

BASIC NUTRITION AND KEY VITAMINS/MINERALS PER SERVING							
Calories	Carbs (g)	Net Carbs (g)	Sugar (g)	Protein (g)	Fiber (g)	Fat (g)	Vitamins/Mineral
200	24	12	6	5	12	8	A, D, E, Calium, Iron

CITRUS SMOOTHIE

Prep Time	5 Minutes
Cook /Chill Time	NA
Cook Temp (F)	NA
Servings	1
Storage	Refrigerate
Storage Duration	1 Day

INGREDIENTS:

1 Grapefruit, peeled
1 Lemon, peeled
1 cup Coconut Water
1 tsp ground Ginger

INSTRUCTIONS:

Combine all ingredients in a blender and blend smooth.

VARIATIONS/SUGGESTIONS:

- Detoxing, healthy liver nutrients/plant fiber
- Super Alkalizing

BASIC NUTRITION AND KEY VITAMINS/MINERALS PER SERVING							
Calories	Carbs (g)	Net Carbs (g)	Sugar (g)	Protein (g)	Fiber (g)	Fat (g)	Vitamins/Mineral
155	35	30	7	3	5	1	C, D, E, Bs, Iron, Zinc

DRAGON FRUIT FROZEN COCONUT CREAM

Prep Time	5 Minutes
Cook /Chill Time	Overnight
Cook Temp (F)	NA
Servings	6
Storage	Freeze
Storage Duration	5 Days

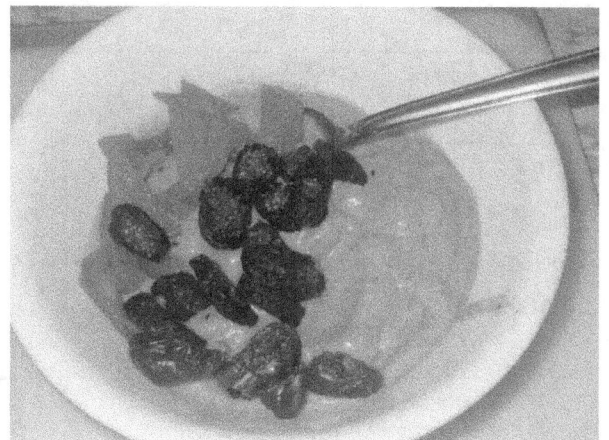

INGREDIENTS:

    1 can Coconut Cream, refrigerated overnight
    ¼ cup Hemp Milk
    1 cup diced Red Dragon Fruit
    ½ cup Pomegranate
    1 scoop Yoli Yes Shake Vanilla

INSTRUCTIONS:

    Scoop out hardened cream from can into blender, storing leftover water for other use. Add the rest of the ingredients and blend into creamy consistency. Ejoy right away or store.

VARIATIONS/SUGGESTIONS:

- Top with sliced fruit/honey/favorite ice cream topping
- Reblend with a bit of milk if it freezes too solid

BASIC NUTRITION AND KEY VITAMINS/MINERALS PER SERVING							
Calories	Carbs (g)	Net Carbs (g)	Sugar (g)	Protein (g)	Fiber (g)	Fat (g)	Vitamins/Mineral
96	16	14	9	3	2	3	C, E, Selenium, Calc.

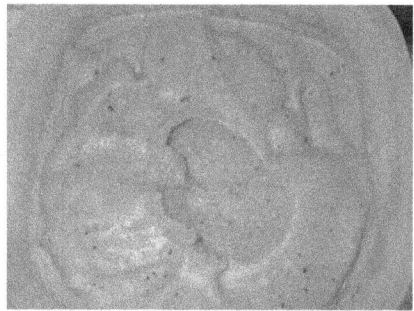
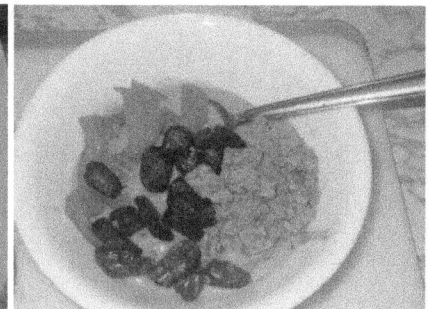

FRUITY VITAMIN SMOOTHIE

Prep Time	5 Minutes
Cook /Chill Time	NA
Cook Temp (F)	NA
Servings	1
Storage	Refrigerate
Storage Duration	1 Day

INGREDIENTS:

1 cup Unsweetened Almond Milk
1 Tbsp Alive Liquid Multivitamin
1 tsp ground Flax
1 tsp Chia Seed
¼ cup Pomegranate
1 Tbsp Unsweetened Shredded Coconut

INSTRUCTIONS:

Combine in a blender and blend until smooth.

VARIATIONS/SUGGESTIONS:

- Add frozen berries for more flavor
- It will be an odd color due to the green of the multivitamin

BASIC NUTRITION AND KEY VITAMINS/MINERALS PER SERVING							
Calories	Carbs (g)	Net Carbs (g)	Sugar (g)	Protein (g)	Fiber (g)	Fat (g)	Vitamins/Mineral
310	28	20	11	5	8	22	E, C, Bs, Mangnesium

ICE BANANA COFFEE MASH

Prep Time	10 Minutes
Cook /Chill Time	NA
Cook Temp (F)	NA
Servings	6
Storage	Freeze
Storage Duration	1 Week

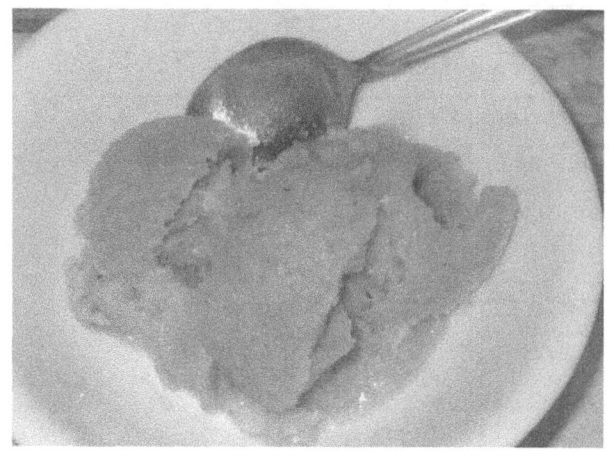

INGREDIENTS:

1 can chilled Coconut Milk Lite
1 scoop Yoli Yes Shake Vanilla
3 ripe Bananas, frozen
1 cup Amaretto Herbal "Coffee"

INSTRUCTIONS:

Mix all ingredients in a blender until thick and creamy. Enjoy or freeze. Blend with extra milk prior to serving if it freezes too solid.

VARIATIONS/SUGGESTIONS:

- Keep in mind bananas have a high glycemic index

BASIC NUTRITION AND KEY VITAMINS/MINERALS PER SERVING							
Calories	Carbs (g)	Net Carbs (g)	Sugar (g)	Protein (g)	Fiber (g)	Fat (g)	Vitamins/Mineral
86	19	16	10	3	3	1	B's, C, E, Potassium

PUMPKIN PIE SHAKE

Prep Time	5 Minutes
Cook /Chill Time	NA
Cook Temp (F)	NA
Servings	1
Storage	Refrigerate
Storage Duration	1 Day

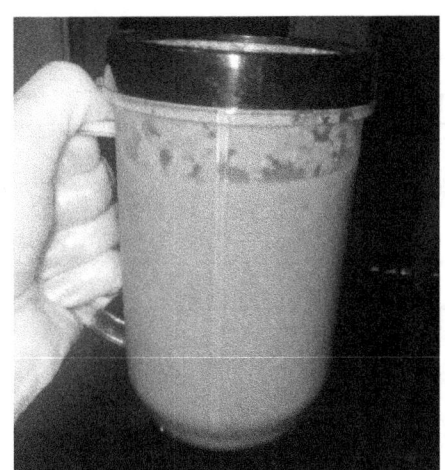

INGREDIENTS:

1 cup Unsweetened Almond Milk
½ cup Pumpkin Puree
1 scopp Yoli Yes Shake Vanilla
2 tsp Cinnamon
1 Tbsp Pumpkin Pie Spice
       Or 1 tsp each cinnamon, giner, clove and nutmeg

INSTRUCTIONS:

Combine in blender.

VARIATIONS/SUGGESTIONS:

• Delicious, healthy pumpkin pie flavor, see also Pumpkin Pie Chia Bowl

BASIC NUTRITION AND KEY VITAMINS/MINERALS PER SERVING							
Calories	Carbs (g)	Net Carbs (g)	Sugar (g)	Protein (g)	Fiber (g)	Fat (g)	Vitamins/Mineral
180	17	11	5	14	6	4	E, Bs, Magnesium

SUPER VEGGIE SMOOTHIE

Prep Time	5 Minutes
Cook /Chill Time	NA
Cook Temp (F)	NA
Servings	1
Storage	Refrigerate
Storage Duration	1 Day

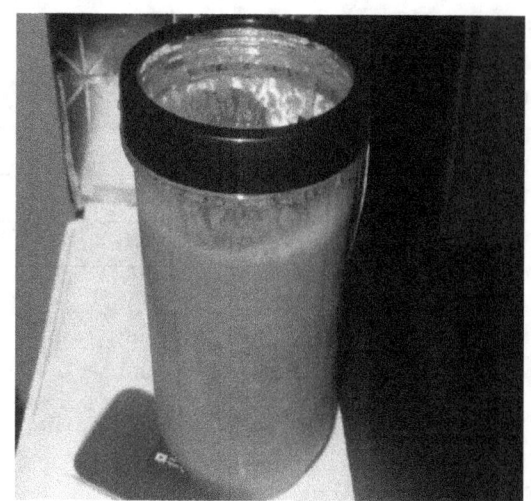

INGREDIENTS:

1 cup Low Sodium Spicy V8
1 cup Baby Greens Mix
¼ cup sliced Cucmber
1 tsp Chia Seed
½ cup Coconut Water
½ a Lemon
1 scoop Super Greens powder
1 Tbsp Alive Liquid Multivitamin

INSTRUCTIONS:

Combine all ingredients in a blender or NutraBullet and blend until smooth. Some blenders will leave strings of the leafy greens if they are not powerful enough or the blades are not sharp enough.

VARIATIONS/SUGGESTIONS:

- Use any veggie juice you like

BASIC NUTRITION AND KEY VITAMINS/MINERALS PER SERVING							
Calories	Carbs (g)	Net Carbs (g)	Sugar (g)	Protein (g)	Fiber (g)	Fat (g)	Vitamins/Mineral
207	39	27	16	8	12	2	A, Bs, C, E, Iron,

Super Low Carb

3 Bean Salad	Pico De Gallo
Alfredo Sauce – Dairy Free	Red Pizza Sauce
Basic Cauliflower Pizza Crust	Savory Veggie Egg Bake
Cajun Shrimp	Simple Egg "Rice" Bowl
Cauliflower Tortillas	Spanish Cauliflower Rice
Egg Muffins	Shepherd's Pie
Garlic Cabbage Rolls	Shredded Mexican Chicken
Garlic Veggie Stock	Shrimp Cakes
Italian Red Sauce	Veggie Cakes
Low Carb Lasagna	Veggie Chili
Low Carb Loco Moco	Veggies Nachos

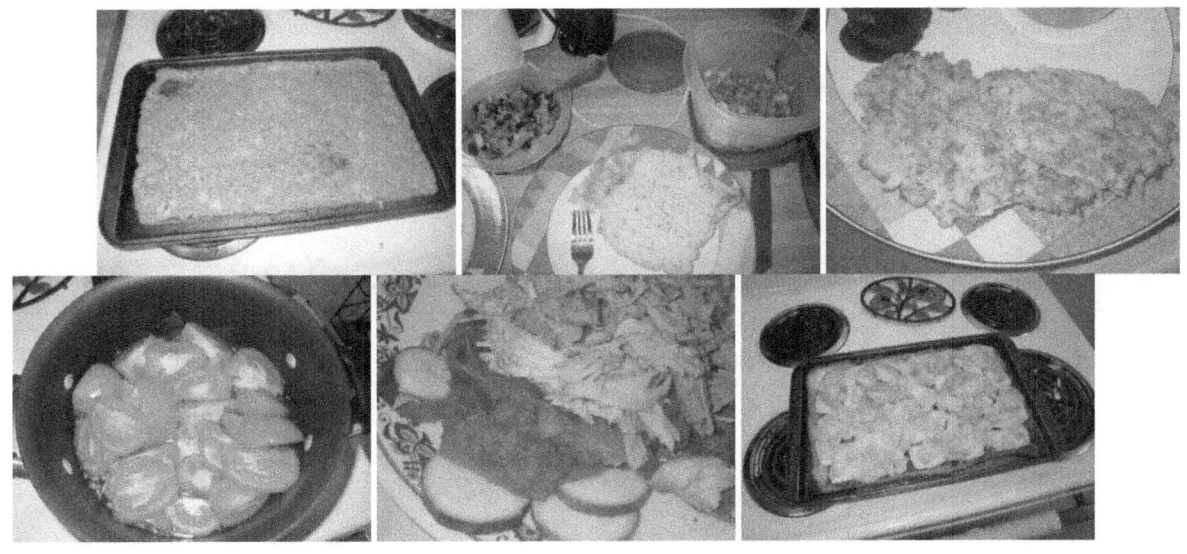

3 BEAN SALAD

Prep Time	5 Minutes
Cook /Chill Time	NA
Cook Temp (F)	NA
Servings	3-4
Storage	Refrigerate
Storage Duration	1 Week

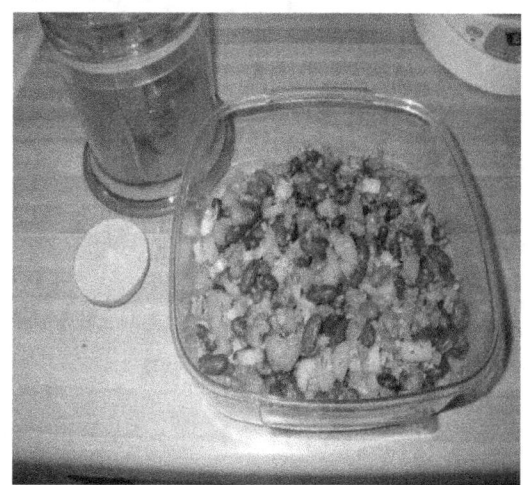

INGREDIENTS:

1 can 3 Bean Mix
5 Celery stalks, diced
1 cup diced Capsicum (any color/mix)
2 Jalapeno Peppers, chopped
1 Onion, red or white, chopped
¼ cup Green Onion, chopped
Juice of 1 Lime
1 Tbsp Parsely, fresh, finely chopped
2 tsp Olive Oil
1 Tbsp Cumin
1 Tbsp chopped Garlic
2 tsp Black Pepper
1 tsp Red Pepper

INSTRUCTIONS:

Toss all ingredients in a large bowl making sure they are well mixed. Chop veggies together in a food processor to mix flavors well.

VARIATIONS/SUGGESTIONS:

- Make the day before serving to allow flavors to meld
- Great for bbq's, pot lucks, etc
- Delicious topping on green leaf salad

BASIC NUTRITION AND KEY VITAMINS/MINERALS PER SERVING							
Calories	Carbs (g)	Net Carbs (g)	Sugar (g)	Protein (g)	Fiber (g)	Fat (g)	Vitamins/Mineral
114	17	8	6	6	9	3	A, K, Magnesium

ALFREDO-ESK GARLIC WHITE SAUCE

Prep Time	10 Minutes
Cook /Chill Time	20 Minutes
Cook Temp (F)	Boil – Med Heat
Servings	2
Storage	Refrigerate/Freeze
Storage Duration	5 Days/2 Months

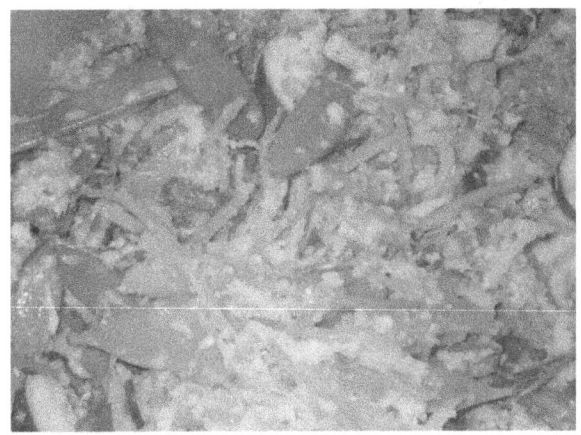

INGREDIENTS:

2 Tbsp minced Garlic
1 tsp Avocado Oil
1 ½ cup Unsweetened Almond/Coconut Milk Blend
1 tsp Black Pepper
½ head Cauliflower, steamed and mashed

INSTRUCTIONS:

Saute minced garlic in avocado oil. Once it browns, add the rest of the ingredients and bring to a boil, then cover and simmer for 20 minutes.

VARIATIONS/SUGGESTIONS:

- Top with Parmesan if you desire
- Great on spghetti squash, chicken, salmon, etc.

BASIC NUTRITION AND KEY VITAMINS/MINERALS PER SERVING							
Calories	Carbs (g)	Net Carbs (g)	Sugar (g)	Protein (g)	Fiber (g)	Fat (g)	Vitamins/Mineral
101	11	9	5	3	2	5	Potassium, Calcium

BASIC CAULIFLOWER PIZZA CRUST

Prep Time	10 Minutes
Cook /Chill Time	40 Minutes
Cook Temp (F)	350
Servings	1 Crust (8-12 pieces)
Storage	Refrigerate/Freeze
Storage Duration	5 Days/1 Months

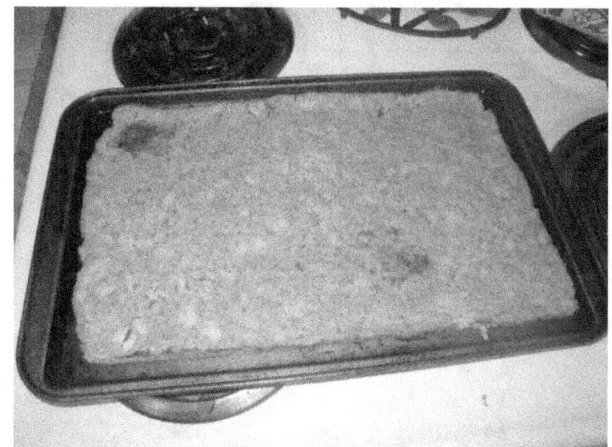

INGREDIENTS:

1 head Cauliflower
½ cup Chia Seed/Flax Blend
1 Egg
Spices to taste (garlic, sage, thyme, basil, etc.)

INSTRUCTIONS:

Steam cauliflower for 5 minutes. In a food processor or blender, chop cauliflower down to flour/meal. Press between papper towels and squeeze out excess water. Preheat oven to 350. Once the meal is mostly dry, combine with the rest of the ingredients. Use wax paper to press meal evenly out in a rectangular pan. Bake for 25 to 30 minutes, flip and bake for 10.

VARIATIONS/SUGGESTIONS:

* Bake at same temperature for 20 minutes after adding pizza toppings
* Add shredded zucchini/finely chopped spinach to give it a veggie boost

BASIC NUTRITION AND KEY VITAMINS/MINERALS PER SERVING							
Calories	Carbs (g)	Net Carbs (g)	Sugar (g)	Protein (g)	Fiber (g)	Fat (g)	Vitamins/Mineral
470	48	16	16	30	32	21	Bs, D, E, Zinc, Iron

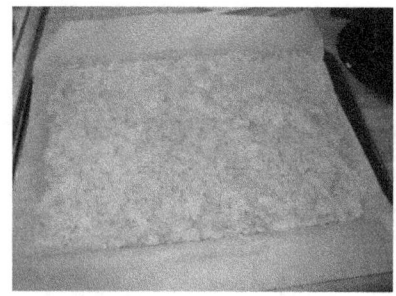
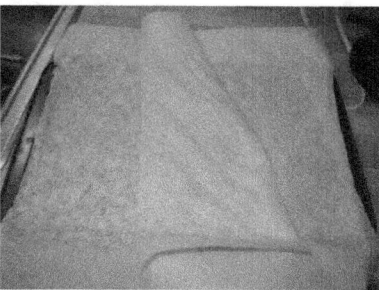
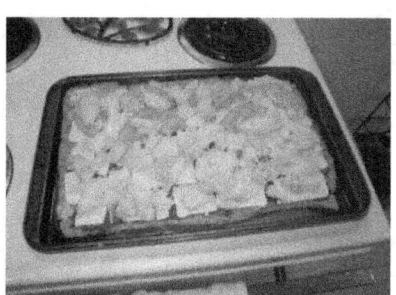

CAJUN SHRIMP

Prep Time	10 Minutes
Cook /Chill Time	20 Minutes
Cook Temp (F)	Medium – Low
Servings	4
Storage	Refrigerate
Storage Duration	3 Days

INGREDIENTS:

1 lb Shrimp, deveined, tail less
¼ cup diced Onion
2 diced Celery Stalks
1 chopped Capsicum
2 diced Roma Tomatoes
1 Tbsp Cajun Spice
1 Tbsp minced Garlic
1 tsp Cinnamon
¼ cup chopped Fresh Parsley
1 sliced Jalapeno

INSTRUCTIONS:

In a non-stick skillet on medium heat, combine shrimp and veggies (minus jalapeno) and cook for 10 minutes, stirring continually. Add spices and parsley and reduce heat to low, cover, and cook another 10 minutes, adding a bit of water if necessary. Use jalapeno as garnish.

VARIATIONS/SUGGESTIONS:

- Add scrambled eggs for a cajun breakfast skillet
- Serve in cauliflower tortillas or lettuve wraps

BASIC NUTRITION AND KEY VITAMINS/MINERALS PER SERVING							
Calories	Carbs (g)	Net Carbs (g)	Sugar (g)	Protein (g)	Fiber (g)	Fat (g)	Vitamins/Mineral
157	9	6	4	25	3	2	Magnesium, Calcium

CAULIFLOWER TORTILLAS

Prep Time	30 Minutes
Cook /Chill Time	15 Minutes
Cook Temp (F)	Medium – High
Servings	6
Storage	Refrigerate
Storage Duration	3 Days

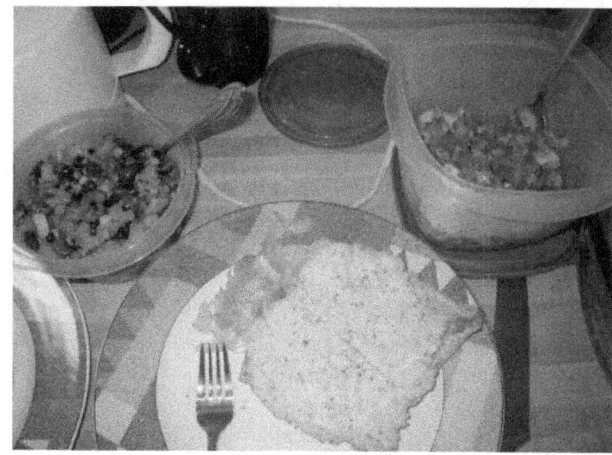

INGREDIENTS:

1 head Cauliflower
2 Eggs
½ cup Flax/Chia Seed Blend
1 Tbsp minced Garlic
2 tsp Black Pepper

INSTRUCTIONS:

Steam the cauliflower for 10 minutes. Let cool and process into meal. Using a clean kitchen towel or paper towel, squeeze out water from the meal. Once the water is mostly gone, mix all ingredients together. Heat a non-stick pan and cook tortillas one at a time, spreading the mixture as thin as possible and cooking 5-6 minutes each side, flipping carefuly.

VARIATIONS/SUGGESTIONS:

- Adapted from a paleoleap recipe
- They may take some practice, don't get frustrated
- Add any seasoning you like

BASIC NUTRITION AND KEY VITAMINS/MINERALS PER SERVING							
Calories	Carbs (g)	Net Carbs (g)	Sugar (g)	Protein (g)	Fiber (g)	Fat (g)	Vitamins/Mineral
103	11	5	4	6	6	4	Iron, Zinc, Calcium

Egg Muffins (mini no crust quiche)

Prep Time	5 Minutes
Cook /Chill Time	20-25 Minutes
Cook Temp (F)	350
Servings	12
Storage	Refrigerate/Freeze
Storage Duration	1 Week/1 Month

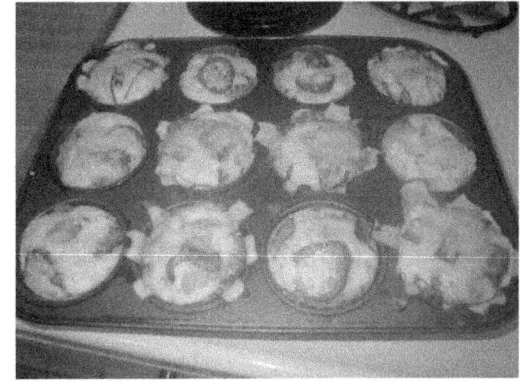

INGREDIENTS:

½ cup shredded Baby Greens Mix
½ cup diced Capsicum (any color/mix)
¼ diced Onion
10 Eggs
3 Tbsp Unsweetened Almond Milk
1 Tbsp minced Garlic
2 tsp Basil

INSTRUCTIONS:

Preheat oven and oil a muffin tin. Place shredded greens and diced veggies evenly into tin. Whisk together eggs, milk, and herbs; pour over veggies carefuly, filling cups about 2/3-3/4 full. Bake for 20-25 minutes.

VARIATIONS/SUGGESTIONS:

- Reheat in oven whenever possible
- Let cool completely before storing
- Yummy cold too
- Top with cheese in the last 5 minutes if you like
- Add flax/chia to boost fiber and healthy fats

BASIC NUTRITION AND KEY VITAMINS/MINERALS PER SERVING							
Calories	Carbs (g)	Net Carbs (g)	Sugar (g)	Protein (g)	Fiber (g)	Fat (g)	Vitamins/Mineral
79	1	1	0	5	0	6	E, Copper, Zinc

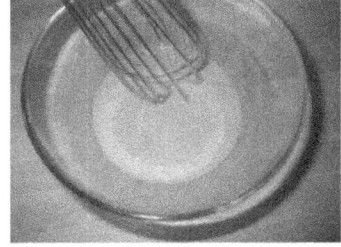
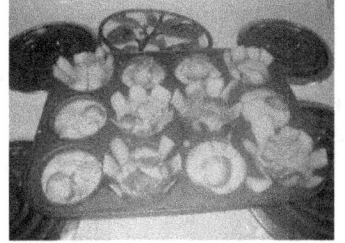

GARLIC CABBAGE ROLLS

Prep Time	10 Minutes
Cook /Chill Time	1 Hour
Cook Temp (F)	Boil – Simmer
Servings	2 (3 Rolls Each)
Storage	Refrigerate
Storage Duration	4 Days

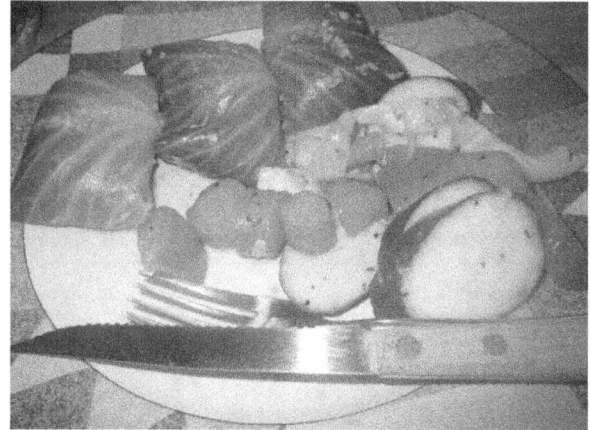

INGREDIENTS:

    6 Cabbage Leaves
    ½ lb Ground Meat
    1 Tbsp minced Garlic
    ½ cup finely chopped Onion
    1 tsp Rosemary
    1 tsp Cinnamon
    1 tsp Black Pepper
    1 cup Garlic Veggie Stock (or water with 2 Tbsp minced Garlic)

INSTRUCTIONS:

In a medium saucepan bring 4 cups of water to boil, add cabbage leaves, and boil for 5-7 minutes. Remove and drain/cool. In a small skillet combine meat, onion, and spices and cook until meat is browned; drain the oil and let cool slightly. Fill the cabbage leaves with 2-3 spoonfuls of meat mixture, fold like an envelope, and place in a saucepan tucked edges down. Pour the garlic stock over the finished rolls. Cover, bring to a boil, then reduce to simmer for 35-45 minutes; cabbage should be fork tender.

VARIATIONS/SUGGESTIONS:

- Use a toothpick to hold rolls together if necessary
- The nutrition for this recipe is calculated using ground turkey

BASIC NUTRITION AND KEY VITAMINS/MINERALS PER SERVING							
Calories	Carbs (g)	Net Carbs (g)	Sugar (g)	Protein (g)	Fiber (g)	Fat (g)	Vitamins/Mineral
217	11	7	4	23	4	8	E, C, Potassium

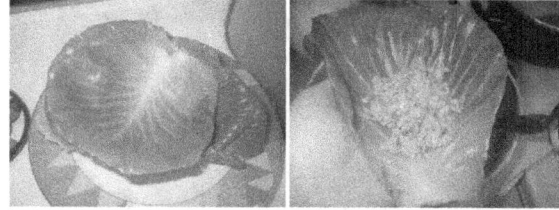 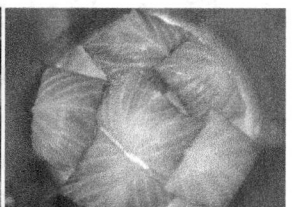

GARLIC VEGGIE STOCK/SOUP

Prep Time	5 Minutes
Cook /Chill Time	30 Minutes +
Cook Temp (F)	Simmer
Servings	4
Storage	Refrigerate/Freeze
Storage Duration	5 Days/2 Months

INGREDIENTS:

3 cups Water
½ cup minced Garlic
8 diced Celery Stalks
1 diced Onion
1 cup finely chopped Fresh Parsley

INSTRUCTIONS:

Simmer all ingredients in a saucepan, covered, for at least 30 minutes. The longer it simmers, the stronger the flavor.

VARIATIONS/SUGGESTIONS:

- An attempt to duplicate the awesome soup they serve in the Czech Republic
- Serve as is with flatbread
- Add smoked meats for a more savory soup
- Use in place of water to add flavor depth to recipes
- Add other vegetables of choice for a clear broth veggie soup
- Strain out the veggies if you only want the broth

BASIC NUTRITION AND KEY VITAMINS/MINERALS PER SERVING							
Calories	Carbs (g)	Net Carbs (g)	Sugar (g)	Protein (g)	Fiber (g)	Fat (g)	Vitamins/Mineral
76	14	8	6	4	6	0	Magnesium, Calcium

ITALIAN RED SAUCE

Prep Time	10 Minutes
Cook /Chill Time	1 – 24 Hours
Cook Temp (F)	Boil – Simmer
Servings	4 Cups or 1 Lasagna
Storage	Refrigerate/Freeze
Storage Duration	5 Days/2 Months

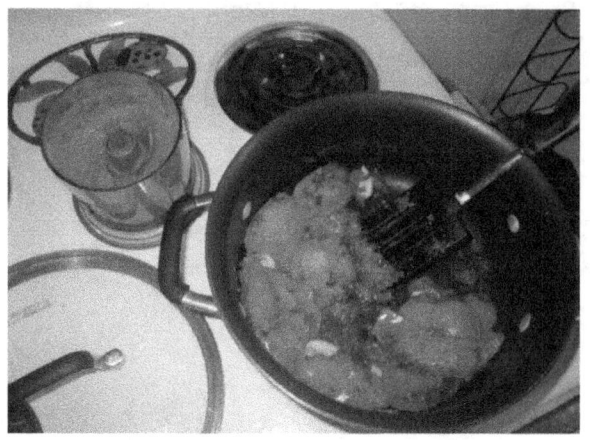

INGREDIENTS:

6 quartered Roma Tomatoes
2 ½ cup Water
1 ½ Tbsp Fresh Basil
6 halved Garlic Cloves
½ cup chopped Onion
1 Tbsp Oregano
½ Tbsp Thyme
½ tsp Rosemary

INSTRUCTIONS:

In a medium pot, place tomatoes, water, basil, garlic and onion; boil for 30 minutes. Remove from heat, pour all ingredients in a food processor or blender and mix smooth. Return to pot, add remaining ingredients and simmer, tasting often and adjusting herbs to taste; the longer it simmers, the better the flavor.

VARIATIONS/SUGGESTIONS:

- Prepare in a crockpot on low to easily let mix 2-24 hours, adding extra water if necessary
- Add mushrooms/meat for a hearty sauce

BASIC NUTRITION AND KEY VITAMINS/MINERALS PER SERVING							
Calories	Carbs (g)	Net Carbs (g)	Sugar (g)	Protein (g)	Fiber (g)	Fat (g)	Vitamins/Mineral
42	9	7	4	2	2	0	A, C, Zinc, Iron

LOW CARB LASAGNA

Prep Time	40 Minutes
Cook /Chill Time	1 Hour
Cook Temp (F)	350
Servings	9 (pieces)
Storage	Refrigerate
Storage Duration	4 Days

INGREDIENTS:

Italian Red Sauce
1 lb Ground Meat, cooked and drained
2 large Zucchini
1 Tbsp Basil
1 Tbsp Oregano
8 oz Ricotta
2 cup shredded Mozzarella
½ cup shredded Parmesan

INSTRUCTIONS:

Mix meat into red sauce and simmer, keeping the sauce fairly thick. Preheat oven. Slice the zucchini lengthwise into about 1/8 inch thick slices. Spread each strip with ricotta cheese and sprinkle with basil and oregano. Place a spoonful of sauce in the bottom of a 9X9 pan. Cover the bottom sith zucchini strips, sprinkle with 1/3 of the cheese, top with 1/3 of the sauce. Repeat. On the last layer place zucchini, sauce, and top with cheese. Sprinkle with herbs and garlic for added flavor. Cover with foil and cook for 45 minutes. Remove foil and cook additional 10-15 minutes, not leting the cheese burn (zucchini should be fork tender).

VARIATIONS/SUGGESTIONS:

- If the sauce is too thick and lasagna looks dry after 15 minutes, add ½ cup of water around the edge
- Nutrition figured using ground turkey

BASIC NUTRITION AND KEY VITAMINS/MINERALS PER SERVING							
Calories	Carbs (g)	Net Carbs (g)	Sugar (g)	Protein (g)	Fiber (g)	Fat (g)	Vitamins/Mineral
252	13	10	5	23	3	16	C, D, Zinc, Calcium

Low Carb Loco Moco

Prep Time	10 Minutes
Cook /Chill Time	20 Minutes
Cook Temp (F)	Medium – Low
Servings	2
Storage	Refrigerate
Storage Duration	2 Days

INGREDIENTS:

2 cup Cauliflower Rice, cooked
½ lb Ground Meat
1 cup sliced Mushrooms
½ cup Thai Kitchen Coconut Milk Lite
1 tsp Black Pepper
4 Eggs

INSTRUCTIONS:

In a small saucepan, simmer together milk, mushrooms, and pepper. After 10 minutes, place in a blender/processor and blend smooth (this is your gravy). Return to heat, adding extra milk if too thick, chia seeds if too thin. Form the ground meat into two patties and grill to desired doneness. Place 1 cup of cauliflower rice on each plate, then the meat patty, then the gravy. Top with 2 eggs cooked however you like.

VARIATIONS/SUGGESTIONS:

- Lower calorie way to enjoy a simple Hawaiin favorite
- Add extra spice to gravy if you like
- I cook my meat to medium and my eggs poached medium
- Nutrition based on ground Bison

BASIC NUTRITION AND KEY VITAMINS/MINERALS PER SERVING							
Calories	Carbs (g)	Net Carbs (g)	Sugar (g)	Protein (g)	Fiber (g)	Fat (g)	Vitamins/Mineral
497	7	5	3	36	2	35	C, E, Bs, Calcium

Pico De Gallo

Prep Time	5 Minutes
Cook /Chill Time	NA
Cook Temp (F)	NA
Servings	4
Storage	Refrigerate
Storage Duration	5 Days

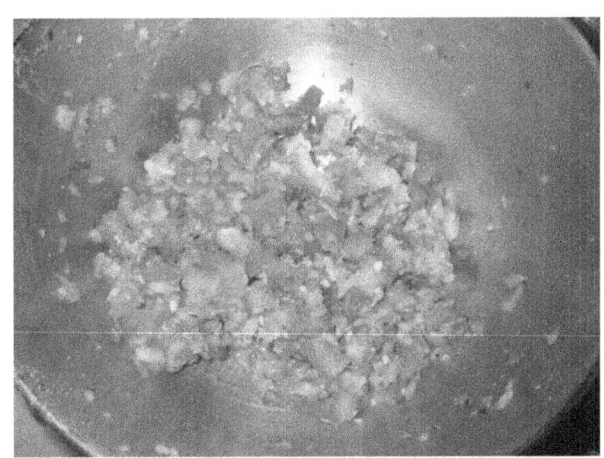

INGREDIENTS:

1-2 diced Roma Tomato
1 diced Onion, red or yellow
½ cup diced Green Onion
Juice of 1 Lime
2 tsp Black Pepper
3 Tbsp minced Garlic
Cilantro to taste

INSTRUCTIONS:

Combine all ingredients in a bowl or food processor. Mix well

VARIATIONS/SUGGESTIONS:

- Add jalapeno to spice it up

BASIC NUTRITION AND KEY VITAMINS/MINERALS PER SERVING							
Calories	Carbs (g)	Net Carbs (g)	Sugar (g)	Protein (g)	Fiber (g)	Fat (g)	Vitamins/Mineral
48	11	9	4	1	2	1	C, Potassium, Zinc

RED PIZZA SAUCE

Prep Time	10 Minutes
Cook /Chill Time	2-8 Hours
Cook Temp (F)	Simmer
Servings	6
Storage	Refrigerate/Freeze
Storage Duration	5 Days/2 Months

INGREDIENTS:

 5 quartered Roma Tomatoes
 1 ½ cup Water
 ¼ cup minced Garlic
 ¼ cup chopped Onion
 2 Tbsp Basil
 1 Tbsp Oregano
 2 tsp Black Pepper
 1 tsp Onion Powder

INSTRUCTIONS:

In a medium saucepan, boil tomatoes, garlic, and onion in water for 30 minutes. Remove from heat and process into paste in a blender or processor. Return to saucepan, add herbs, cover and let simmer for as long as you desire to get ideal taste profile, tasting and adding spice as wanted.

VARIATIONS/SUGGESTIONS:

- Make the night before to really let flavors mix
- Serve on omelettes for a healthy pizza for breakfast spin

BASIC NUTRITION AND KEY VITAMINS/MINERALS PER SERVING							
Calories	Carbs (g)	Net Carbs (g)	Sugar (g)	Protein (g)	Fiber (g)	Fat (g)	Vitamins/Mineral
46	9	7	4	2	2	1	C, E, Iron, Zinc

SAVORY VEGGIE EGG BAKE

Prep Time	10 Minutes
Cook /Chill Time	1 Hour
Cook Temp (F)	350
Servings	12
Storage	Refrigerate/Freeze
Storage Duration	4 Days/2 Months

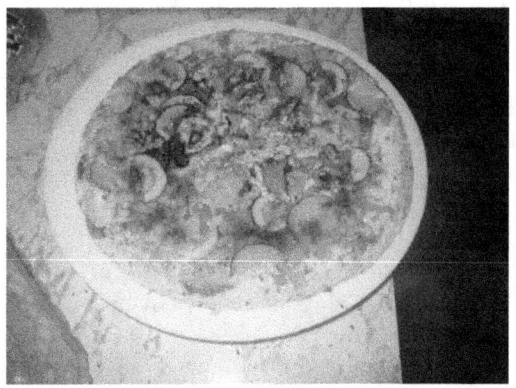

INGREDIENTS:

1 Acorn Squash, partially cooked, peeled, and cubed
¼ cup diced Onion
¼ cup minced Garlic
2 cup chopped Capsicum (any color/mix)
½ cup diced Green Onion
1 cup chopped Asparagus
1 cup chopped Fresh Basil
½ cup chopped Fresh Parsley
2 tsp Rosemary
2 tsp Thyme
1 Tbsp Sage
1 tsp Black Pepper
10 Eggs
Spray Coconut Cooking Oil

INSTRUCTIONS:

Preheat oven. In a 8X12 oiled pan, layer veggies and spices. Whip eggs in a bowl and pour over the top, adding a bit of milk if you wish. Bake covered for 45-60 minutes, until egg is cooked but not brown on the bottom. Let cool 5 minutes before serving.

VARIATIONS/SUGGESTIONS:

- Serve with sliced tomato and avocado for extra flavor
- Add salmon/chickpeas/steak/sausage for flavor and protein
- Add or top with cheese if desired

BASIC NUTRITION AND KEY VITAMINS/MINERALS PER SERVING							
Calories	Carbs (g)	Net Carbs (g)	Sugar (g)	Protein (g)	Fiber (g)	Fat (g)	Vitamins/Mineral
161	18	10	2	8	8	8	E, Bs, Phosphorus

SIMPLE EGG "RICE" BOWL

Prep Time	5 Minutes
Cook /Chill Time	20 Minutes
Cook Temp (F)	Medium – High
Servings	2
Storage	Refrigerate
Storage Duration	3 Days

INGREDIENTS:

1 ½ cup cooked Cauliflower Rice
1 cup shredded Baby Greens Mix
1 Avocado
¼ cup chopped Green Onion
2 chopped Tomatoes
1 diced Zucchini
2 Eggs

INSTRUCTIONS:

In a bowl, layer cauliflower rice, veggies, and top with egg cooked to your taste preference.

VARIATIONS/SUGGESTIONS:

- Add spice to taste
- Add beans/chickpeas/salmon for extra protein and flavor

BASIC NUTRITION AND KEY VITAMINS/MINERALS PER SERVING							
Calories	Carbs (g)	Net Carbs (g)	Sugar (g)	Protein (g)	Fiber (g)	Fat (g)	Vitamins/Mineral
223	12	7	5	10	5	16	E, C, K, Copper

SPANISH CAULI-RICE

Prep Time	5 Minutes
Cook /Chill Time	20 Minutes
Cook Temp (F)	Boil - Simmer
Servings	6
Storage	Refrigerate
Storage Duration	4 Days

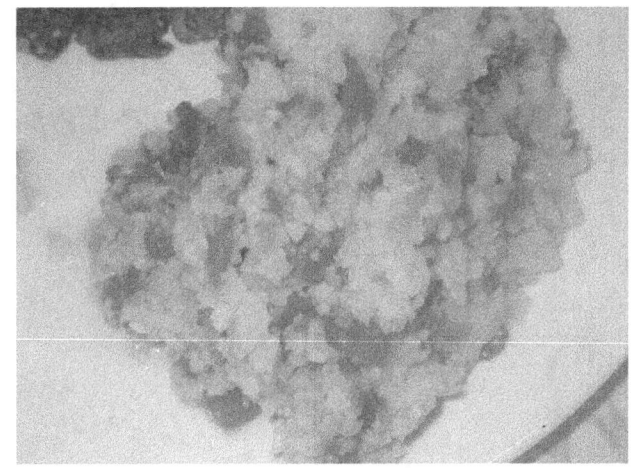

INGREDIENTS:

1 head Cauliflower, processed to rice size
1 cup diced Roma Tomato
½ cup diced Green Chile
1 Tbsp Sriracha
1 Tbsp minced Garlic
1 cup Water

INSTRUCTIONS:

Combine all ingredients in a medium saucepan. Bring to boil, then cover and reduce to simmer. Simmer 20 minutes, stirring occasionally.

VARIATIONS/SUGGESTIONS:

- Serving size depends on size of cauliflower
- Add jalapenpo or chili powder for extra spice

BASIC NUTRITION AND KEY VITAMINS/MINERALS PER SERVING							
Calories	Carbs (g)	Net Carbs (g)	Sugar (g)	Protein (g)	Fiber (g)	Fat (g)	Vitamins/Mineral
40	8	5	4	2	3	0	C, Calcium, Zinc

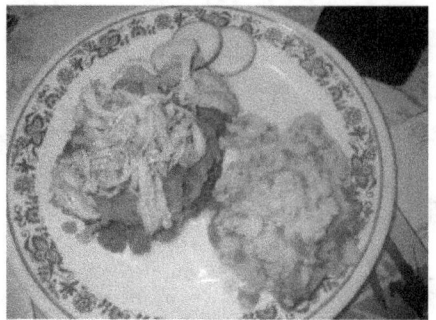

SHEPHERD'S PIE

Prep Time	30 Minutes
Cook /Chill Time	1 Hour
Cook Temp (F)	400
Servings	4
Storage	Refrigerate
Storage Duration	5 Days

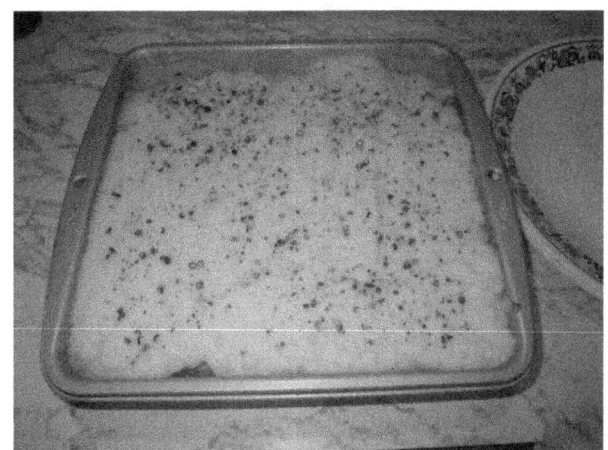

INGREDIENTS:

Red Sauce:

> 4 quartered Roma Tomato
> 1 cup Water
> 1 tsp Tarragon
> 1 tsp Sage
> 2 Tbsp minced Onion

Pie Ingredients:

> ½ lb Ground Meat
> 2 cups Snow Peas
> 1 cup Broccoli Slaw
> 1 cup diced Celery

Mashed Topping:

> 1 head Cauliflower, steamed and mashed with ½ cup coconut milk and 1 tsp avocado oil

INSTRUCTIONS:

Prepare cauli-mash and set aside. Boil sauce ingredients together for 20 minutes. Cook and drain meat while sauce cooks. Pour sauce ingredients in a blender and blend smooth. Preheat oven. Mix sauce, meat, and veggies and pour into a 9X9 pan. Top evenly with cauli-mash. Bake for 20-25 minutes, or until cauli-mash starts to brown. Let cool 10 minutes before serving.

VARIATIONS/SUGGESTIONS:

- Add/replace any veggies you wish
- Add squash/pumpkin to mash for extra flavor

BASIC NUTRITION AND KEY VITAMINS/MINERALS PER SERVING							
Calories	Carbs (g)	Net Carbs (g)	Sugar (g)	Protein (g)	Fiber (g)	Fat (g)	Vitamins/Mineral
225	11	8	5	11	3	16	C, B's, Iron, Zinc

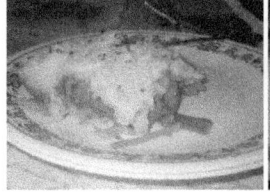 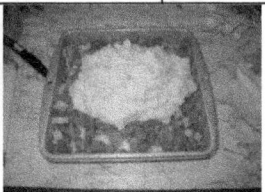

SHREDDED MEXICAN CHICKEN

Prep Time	5 Minutes
Cook /Chill Time	4-8 Hours
Cook Temp (F)	Slow Cooker, Low
Servings	4
Storage	Refrigerate
Storage Duration	5 Days

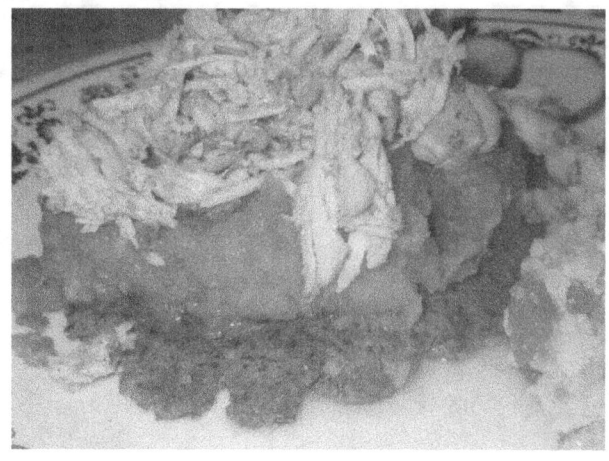

INGREDIENTS:

        1-2 Chicken Breasts
        2 large diced Capsicum
        Juice of 1 Lemon
        1 Tbsp Cumin
        2 Tbsp minced Garlic
        2 cup Water

INSTRUCTIONS:

Combine all ingredients in a slow cooker on low. Cook until chicken is shreddable, shred and enjoy

VARIATIONS/SUGGESTIONS:

- Leftover water can be mixed with mashed squash to make an awesome "bean spread"

BASIC NUTRITION AND KEY VITAMINS/MINERALS PER SERVING							
Calories	Carbs (g)	Net Carbs (g)	Sugar (g)	Protein (g)	Fiber (g)	Fat (g)	Vitamins/Mineral
56	4	3	2	7	1	1	Magnesium, Zinc

SHRIMP CAKES

Prep Time	10 Minutes
Cook /Chill Time	10 Minutes
Cook Temp (F)	Medium High
Servings	6 (small)
Storage	Refrigerate
Storage Duration	3 Days

INGREDIENTS:

2-3 Eggs
1 tsp Black Pepper
2 tsp Sriracha
1 tsp Lime Juice
1 tsp Lemon Juice
1 tsp Ginger
1 tsp Cumin
1 lb Shrimp, grilled and diced
1 chopped Green Onion
¼ cup shredded Zucchini
¼ cup shredded Carrot
½ cup Unsweetened Shredded Coconut
1 Tbsp Avocado Oil

INSTRUCTIONS:

Combine the eggs and spices, whipping until fluffy and well mixed. Fold in diced shrimp, veggies, and coconut flakes. In a large pan, heat avocado oil. Each cake should be one-two spoonful(s) of batter, cooking about 4 minutes each side.

VARIATIONS/SUGGESTIONS:

- Serve with lemon dill sauce for extra flavor
- Make bite size cakes for appetizers

BASIC NUTRITION AND KEY VITAMINS/MINERALS PER SERVING							
Calories	Carbs (g)	Net Carbs (g)	Sugar (g)	Protein (g)	Fiber (g)	Fat (g)	Vitamins/Mineral
185	6	4	2	18	2	10	A, C, E, Bs, Sodium

VEGGIE CAKES

Prep Time	30 Minutes
Cook /Chill Time	10 Minutes
Cook Temp (F)	Medium High
Servings	2
Storage	Refrigerate
Storage Duration	2 Days

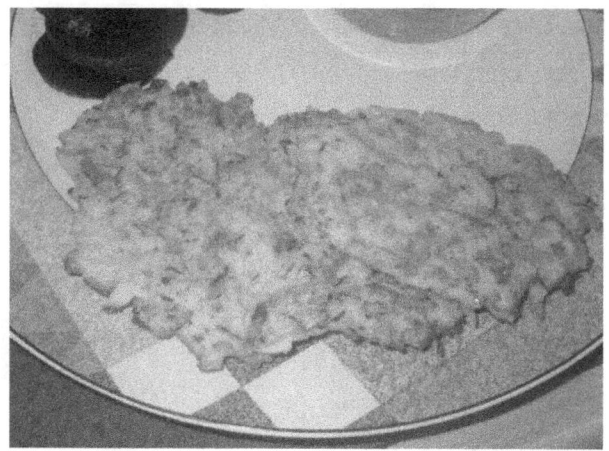

INGREDIENTS:

2-3 Eggs
2 medium shredded Carrots
3 shredded and dried Radishes
3 medium and shredded Zucchini
1 tsp Garlic Powder
1 tsp Basil
1 Tbsp Flax
1 tsp Black Pepper
1 Tbsp Avocado Oil

INSTRUCTIONS:

Shred the veggies and press between towels/paper towels to dry. Combine spices, flaz, and eggs in a bowl, beating until well mixed. Fold in shredded veggies. In a large pan, heat the avocado oil on medium high heat. Spoon four "cakes" into the pan and let cook about 4 minutes each side. Repeat until batter is gone.

VARIATIONS/SUGGESTIONS:

- Add diced onion or celery for a chunkier cake
- Add curry, cumin, and tarragon for veggie curry cake

BASIC NUTRITION AND KEY VITAMINS/MINERALS PER SERVING							
Calories	Carbs (g)	Net Carbs (g)	Sugar (g)	Protein (g)	Fiber (g)	Fat (g)	Vitamins/Mineral
187	10	7	3	12	3	12	A, C, E, K, Iron

VEGGIE ALKALIZING CHILI

Prep Time	10 Minutes
Cook /Chill Time	2-8 Hours
Cook Temp (F)	Simmer
Servings	8
Storage	Refrigerate/Freeze
Storage Duration	5 Days/2 Months

INGREDIENTS:

5 quartered Roma Tomatoes
1 cup water
¼ cup minced Garlic
1 cup Pumpkin Puree
3 Tbsp Chili Powder
1 Tbsp Cumin
¾ cup Thai Kitchen Coconut Milk Lite
2 tsp Cayenne Pepper
1 tsp Cinnamon
1 tsp Allspice
½ diced Onion
2 large diced Capsicum

INSTRUCTIONS:

Boil tomatoes in water for 20 miniutes and blend into paste. Place paste in pot or slow cooker, add the spices, cover and let simmer (or put on low in slow cooker). To avoid overcooking the onion/peppers, add them about 30 minutes prior to serving.

VARIATIONS/SUGGESTIONS:

* Serve over cauli-rice for a yummy dish

BASIC NUTRITION AND KEY VITAMINS/MINERALS PER SERVING							
Calories	Carbs (g)	Net Carbs (g)	Sugar (g)	Protein (g)	Fiber (g)	Fat (g)	Vitamins/Mineral
55	9	6	3	2	3	2	C, Phosphorus, Iron

VEGGIE "NACHOS" - BASE

Prep Time	10 Minutes
Cook /Chill Time	NA
Cook Temp (F)	NA
Servings	2-3
Storage	Refrigerate
Storage Duration	2 Days

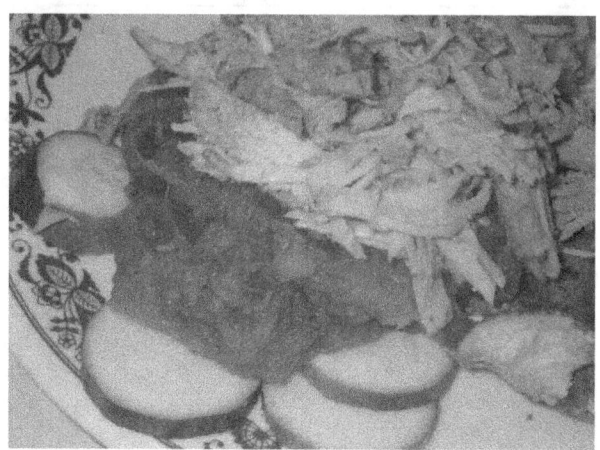

INGREDIENTS:

"Chips":

    2 large Zucchini

"Bean Spread":

    2 Tbsp Tahini
    1 cup Pumpkin Puree
    2 tsp Cumin
    2 tsp powdered Garlic

INSTRUCTIONS:

Slice the zucchini into ¼ inch circular pieces. Mix the "bean spread" and use a knife to evenly spread over zucchini chips. Top with meat, lettuce, tomato, avocado, salsa, sour cream, cheese... whatever you like on your nachos.

VARIATIONS/SUGGESTIONS:

- Nutrition is based on "chips" and spread only.
- Spread mixed with salsa is a great mexican pizza base

BASIC NUTRITION AND KEY VITAMINS/MINERALS PER SERVING							
Calories	Carbs (g)	Net Carbs (g)	Sugar (g)	Protein (g)	Fiber (g)	Fat (g)	Vitamins/Mineral
149	18	10	8	7	8	7	A, C, E, B's, Copper

Anti Inflammatory

Avocado Pesto

Brussel Sprout and Fig Salad

Chewy Protein Bars

Chili Chickpea Squash Bake

Crispy Tofu Bowl

Crockpot Jambalaya

Curry Coleslaw

Fruity Tahini "Rice" Bowl

Garlic Egg Soup

Gingerbread Cereal Squares

Granola Bites

Green Curry

Healthy Country "Potatoes"

Healthy Squash Mash

Marinated Elk w/ Onion-Apple Chutney

Meatball Spaghetti Squash Boats

Mexican Egg Bowl

Mexican "Pie"

Pumpkin Cake-like Bread

Pumpkin Chicken Curry

Pumpkin Hummus Maki Rolls

Pumpkin Porridge w/ Oats

Quinoa Bean Patties

Squash Soup

Superfood Salad

Veggie "Alfredo" Bake

Veggie "Lasagna" Bake

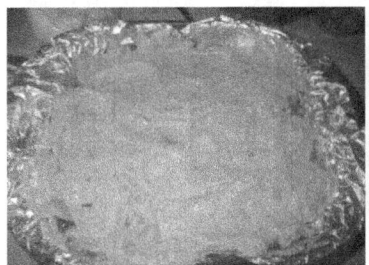 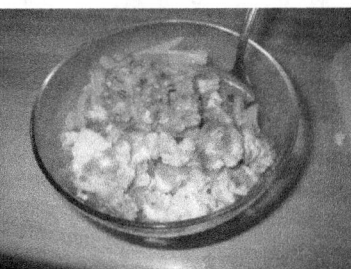 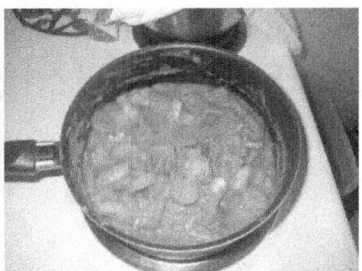

AVOCADO PESTO

Prep Time	5 Minutes
Cook /Chill Time	NA
Cook Temp (F)	NA
Servings	3
Storage	Refrigerate
Storage Duration	2 Days

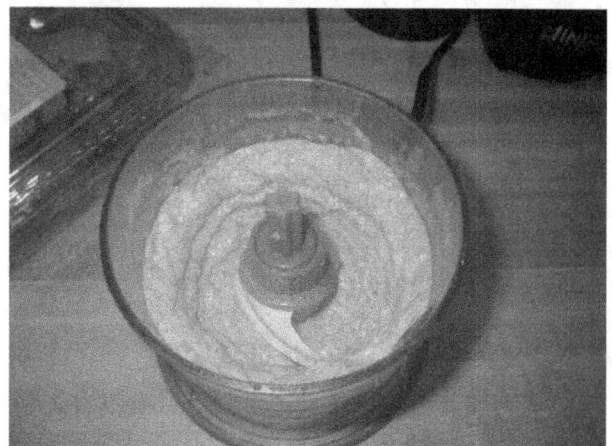

INGREDIENTS:

1 cup Baby Greens Mix
2 Tbsp Basil
1 Tbsp Sunflower Seeds
1 Tbsp Almonds
1 Tbsp Pumpkin Seeds
½ cup Coconut Water
1 avocado
1 tsp Lemon Juice
1 Tbsp minced Garlic

INSTRUCTIONS:

Combine all ingredients in a food processor and blend to desired consistency. Add milk or extra water if necessary.

VARIATIONS/SUGGESTIONS:

- Serve heated over spaghetti squash
- Bake over veggies

BASIC NUTRITION AND KEY VITAMINS/MINERALS PER SERVING							
Calories	Carbs (g)	Net Carbs (g)	Sugar (g)	Protein (g)	Fiber (g)	Fat (g)	Vitamins/Mineral
124	6	3	1	4	3	10	C, E, K, Copper

BRUSSEL SPROUT AND FIG SALAD

Prep Time	20 Minutes
Cook /Chill Time	15 Minutes
Cook Temp (F)	425 / Medium
Servings	2-4
Storage	Refrigerate
Storage Duration	5 Days

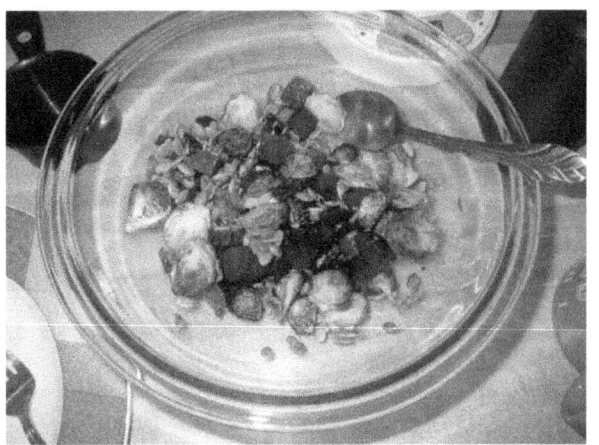

INGREDIENTS:

> 1 cup halved Brussel Sprouts
> 1 cup Beetroor, roasted and diced
> ¼ cup Pumpkin Seeds
> ½ cup sliced Dried Figs
> 1 Tbsp Coconut Oil
> 1 Tbsp thinly sliced Fresh Garlic
> Black Pepper/Spices to taste

INSTRUCTIONS:

In a bowl combine beetroot, pumpkin seeds, and figs. In large saucepan on medium heat combine coconut oil, garlic, and spices. Once the oil is heated and the garlic starts to roast, add the brussel sprouts cut side down. Cook 5-7 minuts, flip and cook an aditional 5-7 minutes (should be nicely brown on both sides). Remove from heat and let cool for 10 minutes. Add brussel sprouts to bowl and toss together.

VARIATIONS/SUGGESTIONS:

- Add nuts, sunflower seeds, other fruit for a broader taste
- Nutrition based on 2 servings

BASIC NUTRITION AND KEY VITAMINS/MINERALS PER SERVING							
Calories	Carbs (g)	Net Carbs (g)	Sugar (g)	Protein (g)	Fiber (g)	Fat (g)	Vitamins/Mineral
311	40	27	23	8	13	15	C, Magnesium

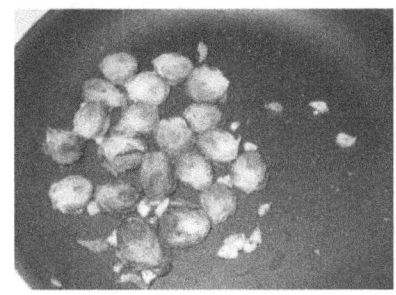 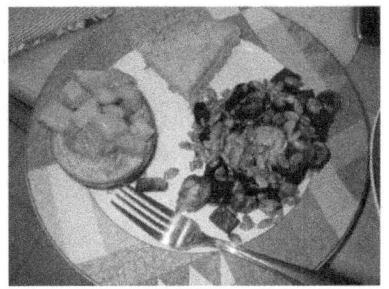

CHEWY PROTEIN BARS

Prep Time	10 Minutes
Cook /Chill Time	30 Minutes /2 Hours
Cook Temp (F)	Boil - Simmer
Servings	20 – 60
Storage	Refrigerate
Storage Duration	1 Week

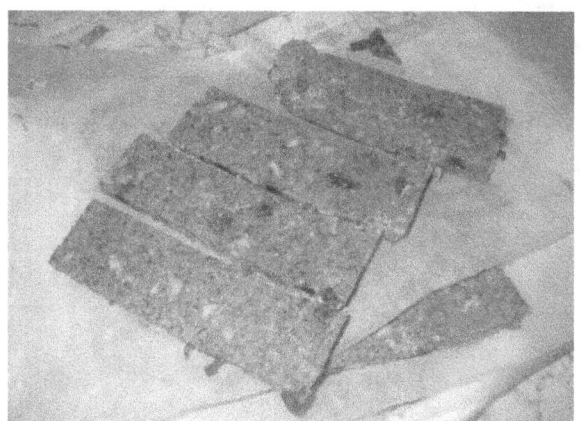

INGREDIENTS:

½ cup Raisins + 1 cup Water
1 Tbsp Cinnamon
1 cup Pumpkin Puree
1 Tbsp Coconut Oil
½ cup Almond Butter
½ cup chopped Unsweetened Coconut Chips
½ cup chopped Pumpkin Seeds
½ cup Chia Seed
1 cup Ground Flax
½ cup chopped Almonds
1 scoop Yoli Yes Shake Vanilla
½ cup Coconut Flour

INSTRUCTIONS:

In a medium saucepan, combine raisins, water, and cinnamon. Bring to boil, cover, and simmer for 15 minutes. Add pumpkin puree, almond butter, and coconut oil, and simmer 10 more minutes, stirring frequently. In the meantime, combine all dry ingredients minuse the coconut flour in a large bowl. Slowly mix in the warmed ingredients; the mix should still be just a little sticky. Add coconut flour a little at a time until it is well mixed but not dry. Spread the mix evenly in a rectangular pan, using wax paper to compress/distribute evenly. Place in the fridge for 2 hours. Remove rom fridge and cut into bars or squares; store in the fridge.

VARIATIONS/SUGGESTIONS:

- Nutrition is based on 20 bars

BASIC NUTRITION AND KEY VITAMINS/MINERALS PER SERVING							
Calories	Carbs (g)	Net Carbs (g)	Sugar (g)	Protein (g)	Fiber (g)	Fat (g)	Vitamins/Mineral
191	14	7	5	6	7	14	Calcium, Phosphorus

CHILI CHICKPEA ACORN SQUASH

Prep Time	5 Minutes
Cook /Chill Time	40-45 Minutes
Cook Temp (F)	375
Servings	2
Storage	Refrigerate
Storage Duration	2 Days

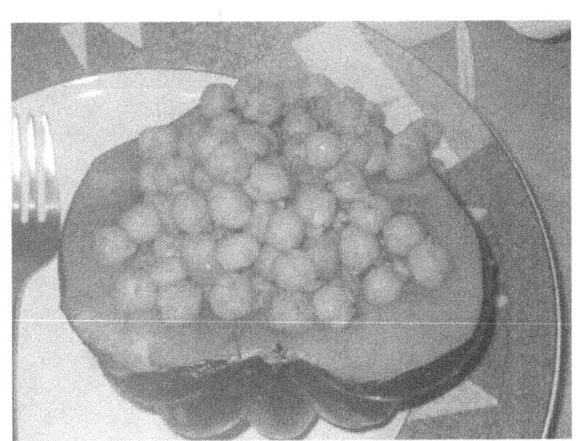

INGREDIENTS:

1 halved, seeds removed, scored Acorn Squash
1 Tbsp Cumin
2 tsp Lime Juice
1 tsp Cayenne Pepper
Spiced Chickpea:
1 can Chickpeas
1 Tbsp minced Garlic
1 Tbsp diced Jalapeno Pepper
1 Tbsp Sriracha
1 Tbsp Coconut Milk

INSTRUCTIONS:

Preheat oven. Sprinkle squash with cumin, cayenne pepper and lime juice. Bake cut side down for 30 minutes. In a bowl, combine chickpeas, garlic, jalapeno, sriracha and coconut milk. After 30 minutes, turn acorn squash over and fill with chickpea mixture (it may overflow, no worries, or halve the can and save some for another meal). Bake an additional 10-15 minutes.

VARIATIONS/SUGGESTIONS:

- Cut down on heat spices if needed

BASIC NUTRITION AND KEY VITAMINS/MINERALS PER SERVING							
Calories	Carbs (g)	Net Carbs (g)	Sugar (g)	Protein (g)	Fiber (g)	Fat (g)	Vitamins/Mineral
271	50	40	5	10	10	6	Selenium, Copper

CRISPY TOFU BOWL

Prep Time	10 Minutes
Cook /Chill Time	30 Minutes
Cook Temp (F)	Low – Medium
Servings	2
Storage	Refrigerate
Storage Duration	2 Days

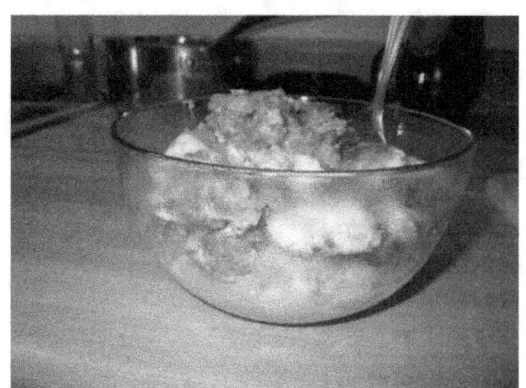

INGREDIENTS:

1 cup cooked Cauliflower Rice

1 package of cubed Tofu
1 Tbsp Coconut Oil
1 medium sliced Red Capsicum
1 medium sliced Yellow Capsicum

2 Tbsp Tahini
2 sliced Jalapeno Peppers
1 tsp Cumin
1 tsp Cayenne Pepper
¼ tsp Black Pepper
4 pitted Medjool Dates

INSTRUCTIONS:

In medium skillet, heat the coconut oil on medium-low. Once the oil is melted add tofu cubes; they should sizzle but not all out fry. Cook the tofu for 7-8 minutes on each side or until all sides have browned nicely. Meanwhile, in a food processor combine tahini, jalapeno, dates, and spices. Blend into a paste. In two bowls, layer rice, veggies, tofu, and top with spicy date paste.

VARIATIONS/SUGGESTIONS:

- Add leafy veggies, broccoli, snap peas etc. for more vitamin/mineral kick

BASIC NUTRITION AND KEY VITAMINS/MINERALS PER SERVING							
Calories	Carbs (g)	Net Carbs (g)	Sugar (g)	Protein (g)	Fiber (g)	Fat (g)	Vitamins/Mineral
461	60	48	40	23	12	19	Potassium, Calcium

CROCKPOT JAMBALAYA

Prep Time	10 Minutes
Cook /Chill Time	6 Hours
Cook Temp (F)	Low
Servings	6
Storage	Refrigerate/Freeze
Storage Duration	5 Days/2 Months

INGREDIENTS:

1 lb cubed Chicken Breast
1 lb deviened, uncooked tailless Shrimp
1 large diced Onion
1 diced Green Capsicum
4 diced Celery Stalks
4 diced Roma Tomatoes
2 diced Jalapeno Peppers
1 Tbsp Cajun Spice
1 tsp Chili Powder

1 tsp Cayenne Pepper
1 tsp Black Pepper
1 tsp Cinnamon
½ cup minced Garlic
1 tsp Thyme
1 tsp Oregano
¼ cup chopped fresh Parsley
2 cups Water
1 ¾ cup Raw Cauliflower "Rice"

INSTRUCTIONS:

Combine all ingredients other than the cauli-rice in the slow cooker. Set on low heat, cover, and cook for 5 hours. Add the cauli-rice and cook an extra hour (you may need to add some extra water).

VARIATIONS/SUGGESTIONS:

- Add sausage of choice for a true Cajun dish
- Use chickpeas in place of the chicken for a more alkaline dish

BASIC NUTRITION AND KEY VITAMINS/MINERALS PER SERVING							
Calories	Carbs (g)	Net Carbs (g)	Sugar (g)	Protein (g)	Fiber (g)	Fat (g)	Vitamins/Mineral
228	16	12	6	34	4	5	C, Magnesium, Iron

CURRY COLESLAW WITH FRUIT

Prep Time	10 Minutes
Cook /Chill Time	NA
Cook Temp (F)	NA
Servings	4
Storage	Refrigerate
Storage Duration	4 Days

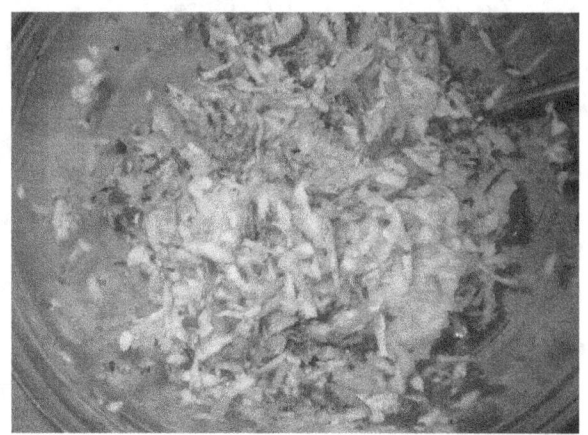

INGREDIENTS:

½ cup Thai Kitchen Coconut Milk Lite
1 Tbsp Curry Powder
1 tsp Cumin
Juice of 1 Lemon
½ cup shredded Red Cabbage
1 cup shredded Green Cabbage
½ cup shredded Carrots
1 shredded Zucchini
1 shredded Granny Smith Apple
½ cup diced Apricot

INSTRUCTIONS:

Whisk spices, milk, and lemon juice together until very well mixed. In a big bowl, combine shredded veggies/fruit. Slowlly mix in curry dressing and toss to mix ingredients.

VARIATIONS/SUGGESTIONS:

- Add nuts/seeds to give it more zing
- Substitute/add fruits you like

BASIC NUTRITION AND KEY VITAMINS/MINERALS PER SERVING							
Calories	Carbs (g)	Net Carbs (g)	Sugar (g)	Protein (g)	Fiber (g)	Fat (g)	Vitamins/Mineral
117	23	18	17	3	5	3	A, C, Phosphorus

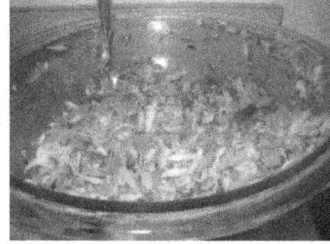
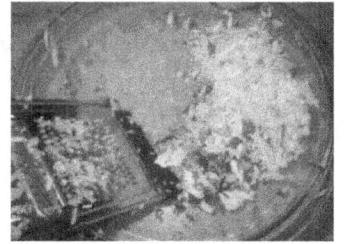

Fruity Tahinini Bowl

Prep Time	10 Minutes
Cook /Chill Time	1 Hour
Cook Temp (F)	400
Servings	2
Storage	Refrigerate
Storage Duration	3 Days

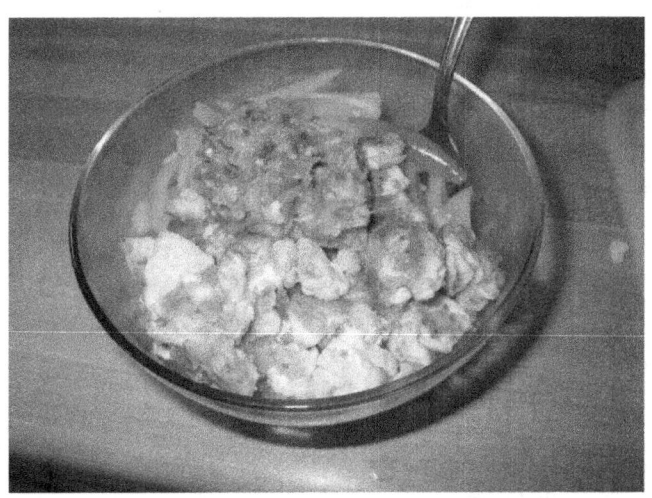

INGREDIENTS:

   1 ½ cup Cauliflower Rice
   1 cup shredded Baby Greens
   1 cup cubed Butternut Squash
   ¼ cup diced cooked Beets
   ½ cup diced Mango
   1 diced Celery Stalk
   2 medium diced Carrots
   ¼ diced Onion
   1 Tbsp Goji Berries
   1 Tbsp Pumpkin Seeds

Dressing:

   2 Tbsp Tahini
   2 Tbsp Thai Kitchen Coconut Milk Lite
   1 tsp Avocado Oil
   ¼ cup No Sugar Added Pomegranate Juice

INSTRUCTIONS:

Preheat oven. In a blender, combine the dressing ingredients, blend well, and store in the fridge. Bake squash for 20-30 minutes and beets until fork tender (about an hour). Cut both into cubes. Make cauliflower rice. In a large bowl combine all ingredients minus the cauliflower rice. In 2 bowls, layer rice, mix, and drizzle with dressing.

VARIATIONS/SUGGESTIONS:

- Add meat or tofu for extra protein
- Add seeds/nuts/fruit for extra zing

BASIC NUTRITION AND KEY VITAMINS/MINERALS PER SERVING							
Calories	Carbs (g)	Net Carbs (g)	Sugar (g)	Protein (g)	Fiber (g)	Fat (g)	Vitamins/Mineral
335	43	8	23	7	9	17	Bs, C, E, Potassium

GARLIC SOUP WITH POACHED EGG

Prep Time	5 Minutes
Cook /Chill Time	30 Minutes
Cook Temp (F)	Medium-Low/Boil
Servings	1
Storage	Refrigerate
Storage Duration	5 Days (without egg)

INGREDIENTS:

1 cup Water
½ cup minced Garlic
2 tsp Black Pepper
1 medium diced Carrot
¼ cup diced Onion
¼ cup diced Celery
1 tsp Parsley
1 tsp Rosemary
1-2 Eggs

INSTRUCTIONS:

Combine all ingredients except egg in a covered saucepan on medium-low heat for 30 minutes. Strain vegetables into a bowl and bring the stock to a boil. Drop the egg(s) in and cook to desired doneness. Spoon the egg(s) on top of the veggies and carefully pour garlic stock over the top.

VARIATIONS/SUGGESTIONS:

- Great for upset tummy days

BASIC NUTRITION AND KEY VITAMINS/MINERALS PER SERVING							
Calories	Carbs (g)	Net Carbs (g)	Sugar (g)	Protein (g)	Fiber (g)	Fat (g)	Vitamins/Mineral
192	24	20	5	10	4	7	A, Manganes, Iron

GINGERBREAD CEREAL SQUARES

Prep Time	10 Minutes
Cook /Chill Time	15- 20 Minutes
Cook Temp (F)	350
Servings	4
Storage	Airtight Container
Storage Duration	1 Week

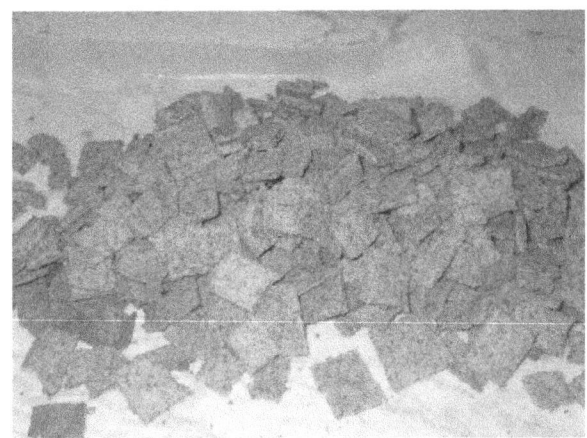

INGREDIENTS:

1 cup Unsweetened Coconut Chips
½ cup Almond Meal
1 Tbsp Ground Flax
1 Tbsp Cinnamon
1 tsp Ginger
1 tsp Nutmeg
2 Tbsp Almond/Coconut Oil blend
1 Egg

INSTRUCTIONS:

Pulse ingreients together in a blender. Roll out between parchment paper to roughly an 1/8 inch thickness. Place bottom parchment paper on a cookie sheet or other pan it will fit on. Score with a knife to desired size. Bake for 10-20 minutes, until it starts to browm. Let cool at least 30 minutes (they will continue to crisp), break apart, and store.

VARIATIONS/SUGGESTIONS:

- Add fruit to jazz it up

BASIC NUTRITION AND KEY VITAMINS/MINERALS PER SERVING							
Calories	Carbs (g)	Net Carbs (g)	Sugar (g)	Protein (g)	Fiber (g)	Fat (g)	Vitamins/Mineral
205	8	3	1	6	5	18	Bs, E, Copper, Iron

GRANOLA BARS

Prep Time	10 Minutes
Cook /Chill Time	2 Hours
Cook Temp (F)	NA
Servings	10-20
Storage	Counter/Refrigerate
Storage Duration	7 Days

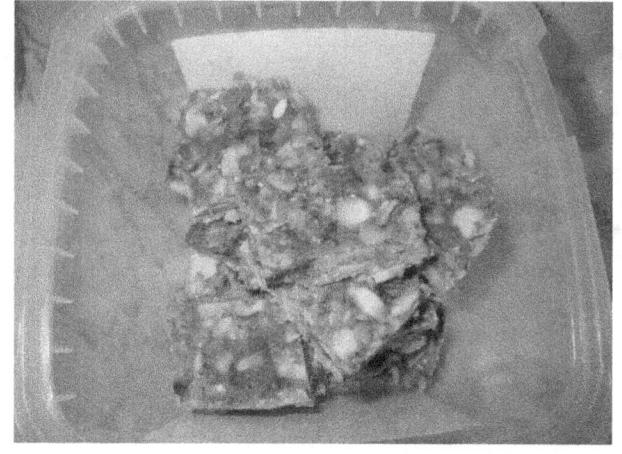

INGREDIENTS:

½ cup Walnuts
½ cup Unsweetened Shredded Coconut
½ cup Sliced Almonds
½ cup Pumpkin Seeds
½ cup Chia Seeds
¼ cup Coconut Flout
1 scoop Yoli Yes Shake Vanilla
½ cup Coconut Oil
½ cup Fig Spread

INSTRUCTIONS:

Make sure nuts and seeds are chopped but not mealed. Combine all ingredients in a bowl. In a saucepan, heat coconut oil and fruit spread on low heat until well mixed. Combine with dry ingredients and mix well. Pour into 9X9 pan and smooth evenly, using wax paper if necessary. Chill for 1-2 hours, cut into 10 granola bars or 20 granola bites.

VARIATIONS/SUGGESTIONS:

- Add dried fruit for extra zing
- Nutrition based on 20 bites

BASIC NUTRITION AND KEY VITAMINS/MINERALS PER SERVING							
Calories	Carbs (g)	Net Carbs (g)	Sugar (g)	Protein (g)	Fiber (g)	Fat (g)	Vitamins/Mineral
148	6	4	2	3	2	14	Bs, D, E, Copper, Zinc

GREEN CURRY

Prep Time	10 Minutes
Cook /Chill Time	30 Minutes
Cook Temp (F)	Low/Medium-Low
Servings	2
Storage	Refrigerate
Storage Duration	3 Days

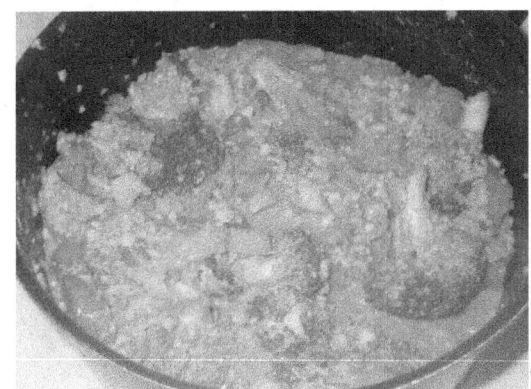

INGREDIENTS:

1 ½ cup Almond/Coconut Milk Blend
½ cup Water
1 Tbsp minced Garlic
1 Tbsp Yellow Coconut Curry Powder
1 tsp Ginger
1 tsp Red Pepper
1 scoop Udo's Powdered Greens
2 cups raw Cauliflower Rice
2 medium chopped Carrots
1 chopped Red Capsicum
1 cup chopped Broccoli

INSTRUCTIONS:

Add all ingredients in a medium saucepan and simmer for 30 minutes.

VARIATIONS/SUGGESTIONS:

- Can be made in a slow cooker for busy days
- Add/remove any veggies you like
- Add meat if you like

BASIC NUTRITION AND KEY VITAMINS/MINERALS PER SERVING							
Calories	Carbs (g)	Net Carbs (g)	Sugar (g)	Protein (g)	Fiber (g)	Fat (g)	Vitamins/Mineral
144	19	12	7	5	7	6	Bs, E, Manganese

HEALTHY COUNTRY "POTATOES"

Prep Time	10 Minutes
Cook /Chill Time	25 + 10 Minutes
Cook Temp (F)	350/Medium High
Servings	2
Storage	Refrigerate
Storage Duration	2 Days

INGREDIENTS:

1 halved, seeds removed Acorn Squash
1 Tbsp Coconut Oil
1 diced Zucchini
¼ cup diced Onion
½ cup diced Capsicum
Spice to taste

INSTRUCTIONS:

Bake squash at 350 for 25 minutes, peel, and cube. In a large pan, melt coconut oil and allow to get nice and hot. Add squash cubes and saute until almost crispy. Add veggies and spices and cook until squash is to desired crispness.

VARIATIONS/SUGGESTIONS:

- Prepare the squash early or the day before to make it easy on you

BASIC NUTRITION AND KEY VITAMINS/MINERALS PER SERVING							
Calories	Carbs (g)	Net Carbs (g)	Sugar (g)	Protein (g)	Fiber (g)	Fat (g)	Vitamins/Mineral
186	25	21	2	3	4	11	Copper, Iron, Zinc

HEALTHY SQUASH MASH

Prep Time	5 Minutes
Cook /Chill Time	15 Minutes
Cook Temp (F)	Medium-High
Servings	2-4
Storage	Refrigerate
Storage Duration	5 Days

INGREDIENTS:

1 cup Pumpkin Puree
4 medium sliced Carrots
½ cubed Butternut Squash

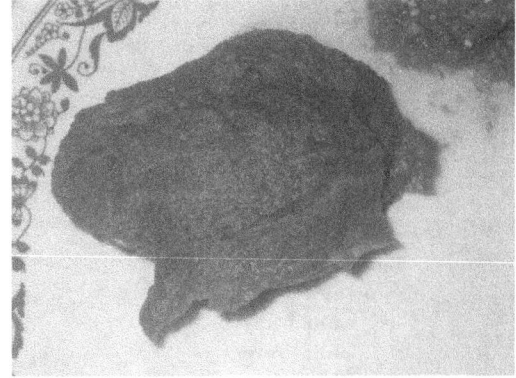

INSTRUCTIONS:

Boil, steam, or roast carrots and squash until tender. With an electric masher. hand masher, or blender mash veggies to smooth consistency, adding in the pumpkin puree.

VARIATIONS/SUGGESTIONS:

- Spice them up with garlic, allspice, etc
- Add pecans and coconut for a healthy dessert
- Nutrition is based on 2 servings

BASIC NUTRITION AND KEY VITAMINS/MINERALS PER SERVING							
Calories	Carbs (g)	Net Carbs (g)	Sugar (g)	Protein (g)	Fiber (g)	Fat (g)	Vitamins/Mineral
117	28	19	11	4	9	1	A, C, E, Iron, Copper

MARINATD ELK WITH ONION-APPLE CHUTNEY

Prep Time	5 Minutes
Cook /Chill Time	40 Minutes
Cook Temp (F)	Medium-Low
Servings	2
Storage	Refrigerate
Storage Duration	3 Days

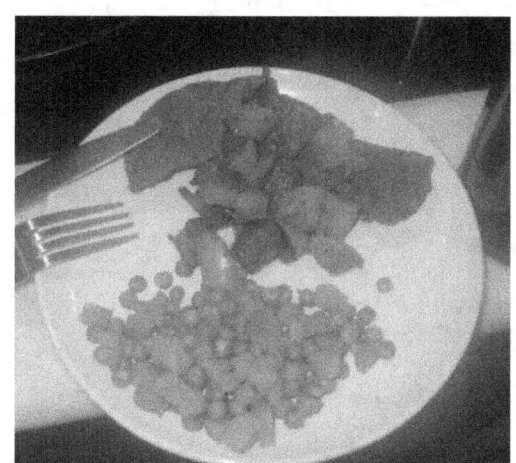

INGREDIENTS:

½ lb thin sliced Elk Steak
1 Tbsp minced Garlic
2 tsp Cinnamon
1 tsp Chili Powder
1 tsp Black Pepper
1 ½ cup Water

Chutney

1 julienne sliced Yellow Onion
1-2 cubed Apples
1 ½ cup Water

INSTRUCTIONS:

Place elk, spices, and water in a container/bag and let marinate. In a small saucepan on high heat, dry saute the onion until it starts to brown; add the diced apple and water. Let boil for 15-20 minutes, mash the apple into an applesauce consistency. Reduce heat to low, stirring ocasionally.

In a separate covered saucepan on medium-low heat, cook marinated elk for 15 minutes each side, water included. Pour water out, turn up the heat to medium high and let dry cook for an additional 2-3 minutes each side. Serve with warm chutney on top.

VARIATIONS/SUGGESTIONS:

• Add sage, basil, oregano for a more herby marinade

BASIC NUTRITION AND KEY VITAMINS/MINERALS PER SERVING							
Calories	Carbs (g)	Net Carbs (g)	Sugar (g)	Protein (g)	Fiber (g)	Fat (g)	Vitamins/Mineral
232	26	21	15	26	5	3	C, Zinc, Iron

MEATBALL SPAGHETTI SQUASH BOATS

Prep Time	20 Minutes
Cook /Chill Time	1 Hour 15 Minutes
Cook Temp (F)	375/Medium
Servings	2
Storage	Refrigerate
Storage Duration	3 Days

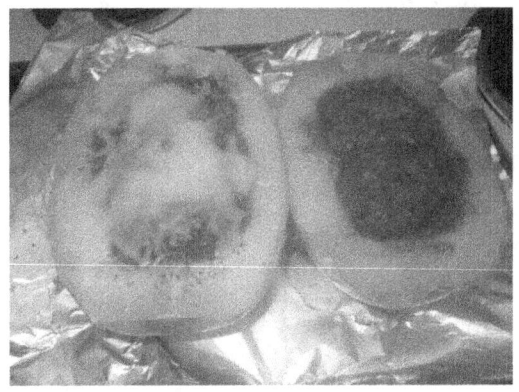

INGREDIENTS:

1 large cut in half, seeds removed Spaghetti Squash
Small Batch Italian Red Sauce:
1-2 large quartered Roma Tomatoes
1 Tbsp Basil
½ cup chopped Onion
1 cup Water
¼ cup minced Garlic
½ tsp oregano
Meatballs:
½ lb Ground Meat
1 Egg
1 Tbsp Ground Flax
Spice to Flavor
1 Tbsp Coconut or Avocado Oil

INSTRUCTIONS:

Make red sauce and let simmer for a few hours. Combine meatball ingredients and form into balls (8-10 depending on size). Heat the oil in a pan and slow fry the meatballs until brown; they may flatten since there is no flour binding them together. Bake the spaghetti squash at 375º for 45 minutes. Reduce heat to 350, turn the squash over, fill with meatballs, top with sauce, and bake for 15 minutes.

VARIATIONS/SUGGESTIONS:

- If you like, top with cheese and cook for 5 additional minutes.

BASIC NUTRITION AND KEY VITAMINS/MINERALS PER SERVING							
Calories	Carbs (g)	Net Carbs (g)	Sugar (g)	Protein (g)	Fiber (g)	Fat (g)	Vitamins/Mineral
429	57	37	16	34	20	15	C, Potassium, Iron

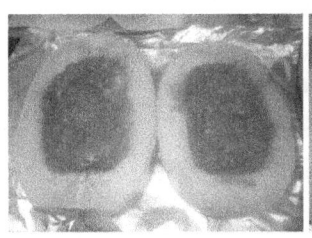 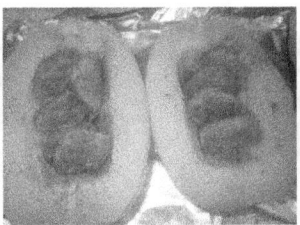 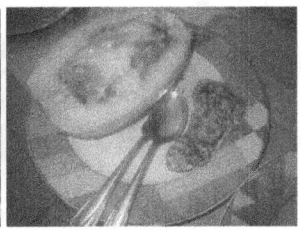

MEXICAN EGG BOWL

Prep Time	10 Minutes
Cook /Chill Time	30 Minutes
Cook Temp (F)	Medium- High
Servings	2
Storage	Refrigerate
Storage Duration	3 Days

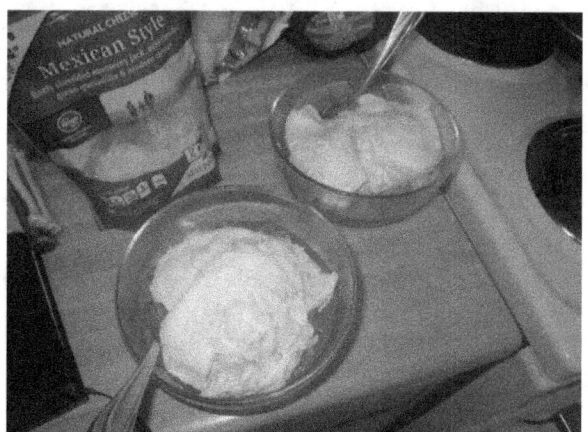

INGREDIENTS:

2 cup Cauliflower Rice
1 cup Water
1 medium diced Roma Tomato
½ cup diced White Onion
1 tsp Cumin
1 tsp Chili Powder
1 can Low Sodium Black Beans
2 medium diced Zucchini
1 cup chopped Baby Greens Mix
4 Eggs, any style
1 sliced Avocado
¼ cup chopped Green onion

INSTRUCTIONS:

In a saucepan bring water, cauliflower, tomatoes, onion, and spices to a boil. Cover and reduce to simmer for 20 minutes. In a small pan on low, heat black beans and zucchini. Prepare eggs to taste. In two bowls, layer rice, greens, bean mix, egs, avocado, and top with green onion.

VARIATIONS/SUGGESTIONS:

- Top with cheese/salsa/sour cream
- Add extra veggies if you like (peppers, etc)

BASIC NUTRITION AND KEY VITAMINS/MINERALS PER SERVING							
Calories	Carbs (g)	Net Carbs (g)	Sugar (g)	Protein (g)	Fiber (g)	Fat (g)	Vitamins/Mineral
508	50	30	9	30	20	22	Potassium, Copper

MEXICAN PIE

Prep Time	10 Minutes
Cook /Chill Time	50-55 Minutes
Cook Temp (F)	400
Servings	4
Storage	Refrigerate
Storage Duration	3 Days

INGREDIENTS:

1 ½ cup raw mealed Cauliflower
1 Egg
1 Tbsp minced Garlic
1 tsp Baking Soda
1 cup Low Sodium Refried Beans
1 tsp Black Pepper
2 tsp Cumin
1 tsp Chili Powder
1 tsp Cinnamon
1 cup Low Sodium Black Beans
1 diced Avocado
1 cup chopped Capsicum
½ cup diced Onion
½ cup sliced Jalapeno

INSTRUCTIONS:

Preheat oven. Mix cauliflower, egg, baking soda and garlic. Spread mixture even'y in a greased/lined pie pan. Bake for 20 minutes, carefully flip, and cook an additional 20 minutes. Meanwhile, in a saucepan on low heat, combine refried beans and spices. Spread mix over crust, top with black beans and veggies, and bake an additional 10-15 minutes.

VARIATIONS/SUGGESTIONS:

- Top with salsa/sour cream/cheese if desired

BASIC NUTRITION AND KEY VITAMINS/MINERALS PER SERVING							
Calories	Carbs (g)	Net Carbs (g)	Sugar (g)	Protein (g)	Fiber (g)	Fat (g)	Vitamins/Mineral
197	25	15	3	9	10	8	C, D, Calcium, Zinc

PUMPKIN CAKE-LIKE BREAD

Prep Time	20 Minutes
Cook /Chill Time	40-50 Minutes
Cook Temp (F)	350
Servings	10
Storage	Refrigerate
Storage Duration	5 Days

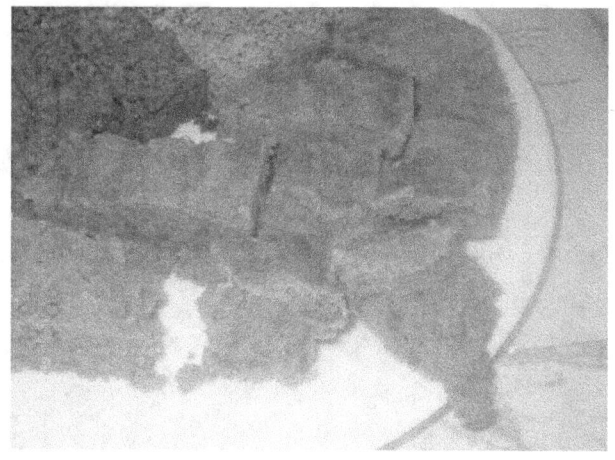

INGREDIENTS:

4 Tbsp Chia
1 cup Water
½ cup Unsweetened Almond Milk
1 ½ cup Coconut Flour
1 scopp Yoli Yes Shake Vanilla
1 tsp Baking Soda

INSTRUCTIONS:

Mix chia and water and let sit for 10 minutes to form egg substitute gel. Miz wet ingredients really well. Slowly stir in the dry ingredients. Spread in a 9X9 oiled pan or bread pan. Bake for 20-30 minutes in cake pan, or 40-50 minutes in a bread pan.

VARIATIONS/SUGGESTIONS:

- Add extra spices as you want
- Top with Coconut Pecan Date Frosting for a yummy dessert
- Add fruits/nuts/seeds to give it character
- Bake as muffind for an easy, on the go breakfast or cupcakes

BASIC NUTRITION AND KEY VITAMINS/MINERALS PER SERVING							
Calories	Carbs (g)	Net Carbs (g)	Sugar (g)	Protein (g)	Fiber (g)	Fat (g)	Vitamins/Mineral
119	15	6	2	5	9	4	B, D, E, Copper

PUMPKIN CHICKEN COCONUT CURRY

Prep Time	10 Minutes
Cook /Chill Time	50 Minutes
Cook Temp (F)	Simmer
Servings	2-4
Storage	Refrigerate
Storage Duration	5 Days

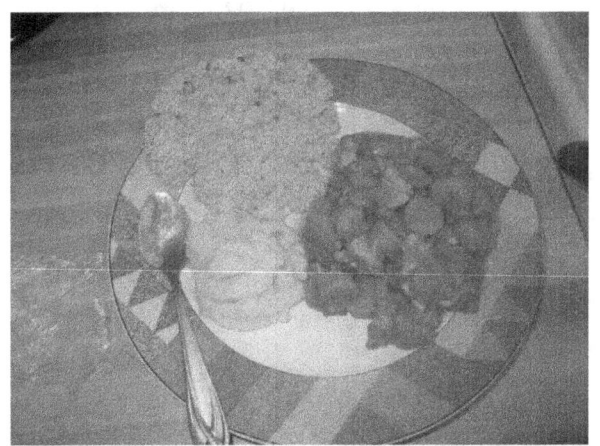

INGREDIENTS:

1 can PumpkinPuree
1 cup Garlic Veggie Stock
½ cup Water
½ cup Thai Coconut Milk Lite
1 Tbsp Curry Powder
½ Tbsp Cumin
1 tsp Paprika
1 tsp Ginger
½ tsp Red Pepper
¼ tsp Cinnamon
½ lb grilled or steamed boneless Chicken
3 sliced Carrots
1 medium chopped Red Capsicum
1 medium chopped Green Capsicum

INSTRUCTIONS:

In medium saucepan, combine all ingredients except the capsicum. Bring to a boil, then reduce to simmer. Simmer for 30 minutes, minimun. Add capsicum 20 minutes prior to serving to avoid over cooking.

VARIATIONS/SUGGESTIONS:

- Add any other veggies/meat you like
- Nutrition is based on 4 servings

BASIC NUTRITION AND KEY VITAMINS/MINERALS PER SERVING							
Calories	Carbs (g)	Net Carbs (g)	Sugar (g)	Protein (g)	Fiber (g)	Fat (g)	Vitamins/Mineral
205	34	19	11	11	15	7	Phosphorus, Calcium

PUMPKIN HUMMUS MAKI ROLLS

Prep Time	10 Minutes
Cook /Chill Time	30/30 Minutes
Cook Temp (F)	350
Servings	3-4
Storage	Refrigerate
Storage Duration	2 Days

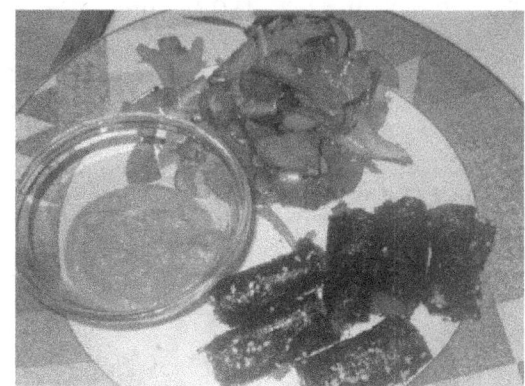

INGREDIENTS:

1 cup Pumpkin Puree
½ cup Garbanzo Beans
1 cup Spinach Leaves
1 Tbsp Sesame Seeds
1 tsp Curry Powder
1 tsp Flax
24 Seaweed Snack Chip Sheets

INSTRUCTIONS:

Combine all ingredients except the seaweed in a blender or food processor and mix into smooth paste. Place in the fridge for 30 minutes. Preheat the oven and line a cookie sheet with baking paper. Using a spoon or Tbsp, place a spoonful of mix into seaweed sheets and roll seaweed around it. Place the rolls on the cookie sheet, tucked edge down, and bake for 30 minutes or until the paste feels firm but not burned.

VARIATIONS/SUGGESTIONS:

- Really fun finger food, great appetizer
- Nutrition is based on 3 servings

BASIC NUTRITION AND KEY VITAMINS/MINERALS PER SERVING							
Calories	Carbs (g)	Net Carbs (g)	Sugar (g)	Protein (g)	Fiber (g)	Fat (g)	Vitamins/Mineral
117	12	9	1	5	3	6	A, C, E, Iron, Copper

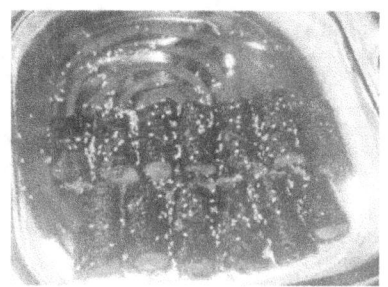

PUMPKIN PORRIDGE WITH OATS

Prep Time	5 Minutes
Cook /Chill Time	15 Minutes
Cook Temp (F)	Simmer
Servings	1
Storage	Refrigerate
Storage Duration	2 Days

INGREDIENTS:

½ cup Pumpkin Puree
½ cup Oats of choice
½ cup Thai Kitchen Coconut Milk Lite
1 Tbsp Cinnamon

INSTRUCTIONS:

Combine all ingredients in a small saucepan. Mix and let simmer for 15 minutes.

VARIATIONS/SUGGESTIONS:

- Omit oats for a yummy, simple breakfast "soup"

BASIC NUTRITION AND KEY VITAMINS/MINERALS PER SERVING							
Calories	Carbs (g)	Net Carbs (g)	Sugar (g)	Protein (g)	Fiber (g)	Fat (g)	Vitamins/Mineral
253	39	24	7	7	15	10	Bs, C, E, Magnesium

QUINOA BEAN PATTIES

Prep Time	10 Minutes
Cook /Chill Time	30/30 Minutes
Cook Temp (F)	375
Servings	6
Storage	Refrigerate
Storage Duration	5 Days

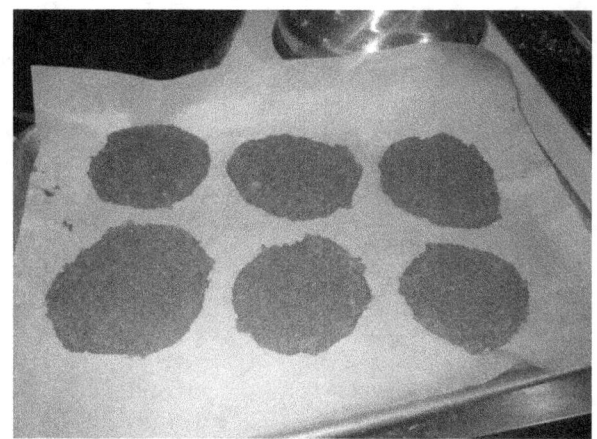

INGREDIENTS:

1 cup Low Sodium Chickpeas
1 cup Baby Greens Mix
1 cup Low Sodium Black Beans
½ cup chopped Onion
½ cup chopped Parsley
½ cup cooked Quinoa
¼ cup minced Garlic
1 Tbsp Lemon Juice
1 Tbsp Sesame Seeds
1 tsp Flax
1 tsp Black Pepper
1 tsp Ginger
½ tsp Black Pepper

INSTRUCTIONS:

Combine all ingredients in a food processor into a paste. Let sit in the fridge for 30 minutes. Preheat oven. Form batter into 6 patties and place on a cookie sheet lined with baking paper. Bake for 30 minutes or until patties start to brown. Let sit 10 minutes before serving.

VARIATIONS/SUGGESTIONS:

- Wrap in lettuce with tomato and avocado
- Top with lemon dill or kefir dill sauce for added zing

BASIC NUTRITION AND KEY VITAMINS/MINERALS PER SERVING							
Calories	Carbs (g)	Net Carbs (g)	Sugar (g)	Protein (g)	Fiber (g)	Fat (g)	Vitamins/Mineral
169	30	22	1	9	8	2	Magnesium, Zinc

SQUASH SOUP - BASE

Prep Time	5 Minutes
Cook /Chill Time	10 Minutes
Cook Temp (F)	Medium
Servings	4-6
Storage	Refrigerate/Freeze
Storage Duration	5 Days/2 Months

INGREDIENTS:

1 can Pumpkin Puree
2 cup mashed Butternut Squash
6 medium cooked and mashed Carrots
1 cup Thai Kitchen Coconut Milk Lite
2 cup Water
1 tsp Black Pepper

INSTRUCTIONS:

Mix all ingredients in a saucepan and heat.

VARIATIONS/SUGGESTIONS:

- Add sliced veggies/meat/spices of choice or enjoy on it's own
- Serve with Flax Flatbread
- Nutrition based on 6 servings

BASIC NUTRITION AND KEY VITAMINS/MINERALS PER SERVING							
Calories	Carbs (g)	Net Carbs (g)	Sugar (g)	Protein (g)	Fiber (g)	Fat (g)	Vitamins/Mineral
133	32	19	9	6	13	8	A, C, E, Calcium, Iron

SUPERFOOD SALAD

Prep Time	5 Minutes
Cook /Chill Time	NA
Cook Temp (F)	NA
Servings	4
Storage	Refrigerate
Storage Duration	2 Days

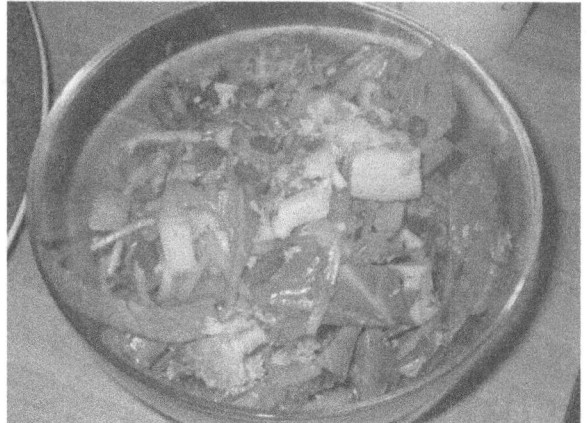

INGREDIENTS:

2 cup Power Greens Mix
1 medium shredded Carrot
4 chopped Celery Stalks
1 diced Cucumber
1 diced Avocado
½ cup chopped Broccoli
½ cup diced Red Onion
1 Tbsp Pumpkin Seeds
1 Tbsp Ground Flax
1 Tbsp Walnut Halves
1 Tbsp Sliced Almonds
1 Tbsp Goji Berries
2 tsp Sunflower Seeds

Dressing:
1 Tbsp Avocado/Coconut Oil Blend
¼ cup Pomegranate
2 tsp Lemon Juice
1 tsp Grapefruit Juice

INSTRUCTIONS:

Mix pomegranates with juice and oil. In big salad bowl combine salad ingredients. Toss with dressing.

VARIATIONS/SUGGESTIONS:

- Jazz it up with herbs

BASIC NUTRITION AND KEY VITAMINS/MINERALS PER SERVING							
Calories	Carbs (g)	Net Carbs (g)	Sugar (g)	Protein (g)	Fiber (g)	Fat (g)	Vitamins/Mineral
182	18	12	8	5	6	12	Bs, E, K, Copper

VEGGIE ALFREDO-ESK BAKE

Prep Time	10 Minutes
Cook /Chill Time	45-55 Minutes
Cook Temp (F)	375
Servings	3
Storage	Refrigerate
Storage Duration	2 Days

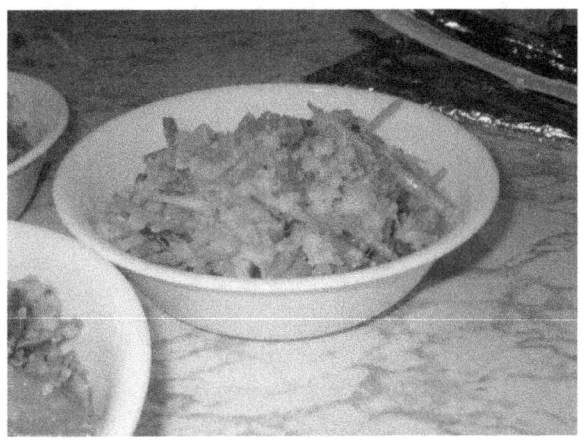

INGREDIENTS:

White Sauce:

> 1 ½ cup Almond/Coconut Milk Blend
> 2 Tbsp minced Garlic
> 1 tsp Avocado Oil
> 1 tsp Black Pepper

Veggies:

> 1 cup Broccoli Slaw
> 1 cup Power Greens Mix
> ½ cup Snow Peas
> ½ cup Alfalfa Sprouts
> 1 sliced Zucchini

INSTRUCTIONS:

In a medium saucepane, saute garlic in oil until it starts to brown. Add milk and pepper and simmer together for 15 minutes. Place veggies into a 9X9 pan, top with white sauce and bake covered for 30-40 minutes. Veggies will lose waer so stir a few times while cooking to ensure the veggies are evenly coated.

VARIATIONS/SUGGESTIONS:

- Add meat to make it more hearty
- Serve as a side dish or main

BASIC NUTRITION AND KEY VITAMINS/MINERALS PER SERVING							
Calories	Carbs (g)	Net Carbs (g)	Sugar (g)	Protein (g)	Fiber (g)	Fat (g)	Vitamins/Mineral
171	18	14	8	5	4	9	Bs, E, Copper, Sodium

VEGGIE LASAGNA-ESK BAKE

Prep Time	20 Minutes
Cook /Chill Time	1 Hour
Cook Temp (F)	375
Servings	9 Pieces
Storage	Refrigerate
Storage Duration	4 Days

INGREDIENTS:

Italian Red Sauce
2 cup Sliced Mushrooms
2 medium diced Capsicum
2 Zucchini, sliced lengthwise into noodles
1 can Pumpkin Puree
4 baked and mashed Carrots
2 cups mashed Acorn Squash

INSTRUCTIONS:

Make italian red sauce and add capsicum and mushrooms. Blend together pumpkin, carrots, and acorn squash. Spoon a small amount of sauce into the bottom of a 9X9 pan and coat. Layer zucchini noodles, mash, and sauce, repeat until pan is full and top with the zucchini slices. Cover and bake for 40 minutes. Remove foil and bake an additional 15 minutes, or until zucchini is fork tender.

VARIATIONS/SUGGESTIONS:

- Make sauce thick as zucchini are full of water
- Carefully drain excess water as necessary
- Add eggplant for extra layer/flavor

BASIC NUTRITION AND KEY VITAMINS/MINERALS PER SERVING							
Calories	Carbs (g)	Net Carbs (g)	Sugar (g)	Protein (g)	Fiber (g)	Fat (g)	Vitamins/Mineral
96	20	15	7	4	5	2	C, E, Phosphorus

Omega Power

Almond Butter Chia Bowl

Apple Pie Chia Pudding

Avocado Chocolate Pudding

Avocado Lime Pudding

Chocolate Avocado Protein Cookies

Cinnamon Roll Chia Pudding

Egg Baked Avocado

Flax Flatbread

Fourth of July Chia Parfaits

Guacomole

Lemon Pie Chia Pudding

Lime Pie Chia Pudding

Lox "Rice" Bowl

Mexican Mocha Chia Pudding

No Mayo Chicken Salad

No Mayo Egg Salad

Pecan Pie Chia Pudding

Pumpkin Pie Chia Pudding

Salmon Baked Avocado

Shrimp Stuffed Avocado

Spicy Salmon Aton Spaghetti Squash

Sunflower Soda Bread

Tuna Bruschetta Patties

Vanilla Protein Flax Cereal

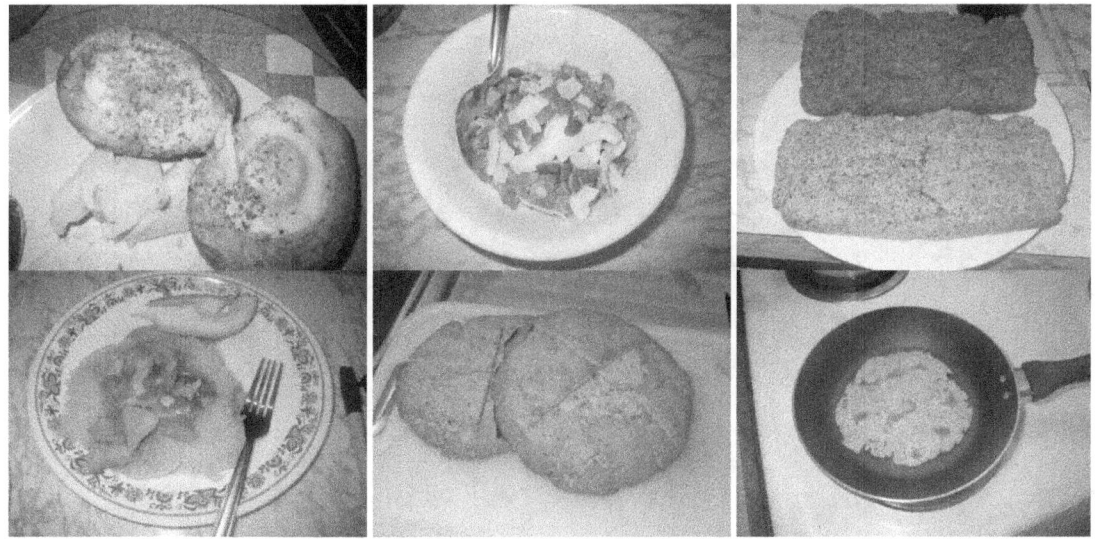

ALMOND BUTTER CHIA BOWL

Prep Time	5 Minutes
Cook /Chill Time	2 Hours/Overnight
Cook Temp (F)	NA
Servings	2
Storage	Refrigerate
Storage Duration	2 Days

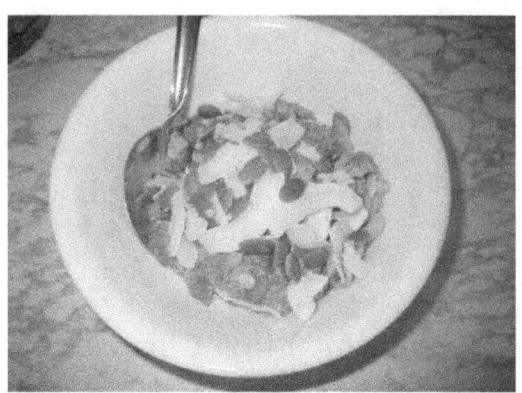

INGREDIENTS:

1 cup Unsweetened Almond Milk
2 Tbsp Almond Butter
2 Tbsp Chia Seed
½ scoop Yoli Yes Shake Vanilla

INSTRUCTIONS:

Mix and chill at least 2 hours.

VARIATIONS/SUGGESTIONS:

- Use chocolate Shake if desired
- Top with granola/fruit/nuts/seeds

BASIC NUTRITION AND KEY VITAMINS/MINERALS PER SERVING							
Calories	Carbs (g)	Net Carbs (g)	Sugar (g)	Protein (g)	Fiber (g)	Fat (g)	Vitamins/Mineral
184	10	2	1	7	8	15	D, Calcium, Copper

APPLE PIE CHIA PUDDING

Prep Time	5 Minutes
Cook /Chill Time	2 Hours/Overnight
Cook Temp (F)	NA
Servings	2
Storage	Refrigerate
Storage Duration	2 Days

INGREDIENTS:

1 ½ cup Unsweetened Almond Milk
½ cup no sugar addded Apple Butter or Applesauce
3 Tbsp Chia Seeds
1 Tbsp Almond Butter
2 tsp Cinnamon
1 tsp Nutmeg
1 tsp Ground Flax

INSTRUCTIONS:

Mix all ingredients in a blender and chill at least 2 hours.

VARIATIONS/SUGGESTIONS:

- Add vanilla protein powder for protein kick
- Top with finely chopped seeds/nuts for crust like crunch

BASIC NUTRITION AND KEY VITAMINS/MINERALS PER SERVING							
Calories	Carbs (g)	Net Carbs (g)	Sugar (g)	Protein (g)	Fiber (g)	Fat (g)	Vitamins/Mineral
335	45	31	25	9	14	14	Magnesium, Copper

AVOCADO CHOCOLATE PUDDING

Prep Time	5 Minutes
Cook /Chill Time	NA
Cook Temp (F)	NA
Servings	4
Storage	Refrigerate
Storage Duration	2 Days

INGREDIENTS:

2 Avocado
3 Tbsp Cocoa Powder or Chocolate Protein Powder
¼ cup fresh Blueberries
1 Tbsp Thai Lite Coconut Milk

INSTRUCTIONS:

Combine all ingredients in a food processor and blend until creamy

VARIATIONS/SUGGESTIONS:

- Adapted from a Food Matters recipe
- Add cinnamon or chili powder to spice it up
- Top with gojie berries for a superfood kick

BASIC NUTRITION AND KEY VITAMINS/MINERALS PER SERVING							
Calories	Carbs (g)	Net Carbs (g)	Sugar (g)	Protein (g)	Fiber (g)	Fat (g)	Vitamins/Mineral
130	20	14	10	2	6	7	K, Potassium, Iron

AVOCADO LIME PUDDING

Prep Time	5 Minutes
Cook /Chill Time	NA
Cook Temp (F)	NA
Servings	4
Storage	Refrigerate
Storage Duration	3 Days

INGREDIENTS:

2 Avocado
4 peeled Limes
2 scoops Yoli Yes Shake Vanilla

INSTRUCTIONS:

Combine all ingredients in a blender and blend smooth. Can be served right away or chilled for later

VARIATIONS/SUGGESTIONS:

* Top with nuts/whipped coconut cream for a great dessert

BASIC NUTRITION AND KEY VITAMINS/MINERALS PER SERVING							
Calories	Carbs (g)	Net Carbs (g)	Sugar (g)	Protein (g)	Fiber (g)	Fat (g)	Vitamins/Mineral
127	12	8	2	6	4	8	C, E, Copper

CHOCOLATE AVOCADO PROTEIN COOKIES

Prep Time	5 Minutes
Cook /Chill Time	10-15 Minutes
Cook Temp (F)	350
Servings	4
Storage	Air Tight Container
Storage Duration	6 Days

INGREDIENTS:

1 Avocado
½ cup Steele Cut Oats
1 Tbsp Almond Butter
1 Tbsp Unsweetened Shredded Coconut
2 tsp Flax
2 tsp Chia
2 tsp Cinnamon
2 scoop Yoli Yes Shake Chocolate

INSTRUCTIONS:

Preheat oven. In a blender, combine all ingredients, dough will be faitly thick. On a lined or oiled cookie sheet, form four cookies, or roll into bite size balls, and bake

VARIATIONS/SUGGESTIONS:

- Perfect recipe for a sweet protein treat without overstock
- Sub any nut/seed butter you like
- Sub banana if you really don't like avocado
- Sub coconut oil for shredded coconut if you wish

BASIC NUTRITION AND KEY VITAMINS/MINERALS PER SERVING							
Calories	Carbs (g)	Net Carbs (g)	Sugar (g)	Protein (g)	Fiber (g)	Fat (g)	Vitamins/Mineral
166	8	9	2	9	7	8	Bs, C, E, Copper

CINNAMON ROLL CHIA PROTEIN PUDDING

Prep Time	5 Minutes
Cook /Chill Time	2 Hours
Cook Temp (F)	NA
Servings	2
Storage	Refrigerate
Storage Duration	2 Days

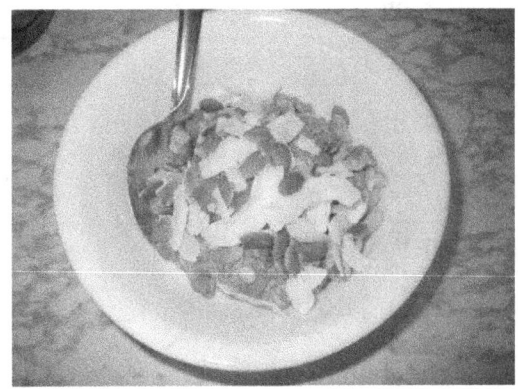

INGREDIENTS:

1 cup Unsweetened Almond Milk
1 scoop Yoli Yes Shake Vanilla
2 Tbsp Chia Seed
2 tsp Cinnamon

INSTRUCTIONS:

Mix all ingredients and refrigerate for 2 hours minimum.

VARIATIONS/SUGGESTIONS:

- Because it has cinnamon, overnight is best
- Great topped with nuts/raisins.coconut

BASIC NUTRITION AND KEY VITAMINS/MINERALS PER SERVING							
Calories	Carbs (g)	Net Carbs (g)	Sugar (g)	Protein (g)	Fiber (g)	Fat (g)	Vitamins/Mineral
126	13	4	2	9	9	7	

Egg Baked Avocado

Prep Time	5 Minutes
Cook /Chill Time	15 Minutes
Cook Temp (F)	425
Servings	2
Storage	Refrigerate
Storage Duration	1 Day

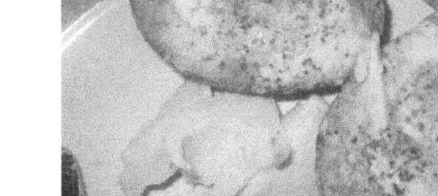

INGREDIENTS:

2 Avocado
4 Eggs
Spices of Choice (pepper, garlic, basil, sage, etc)

INSTRUCTIONS:

Preheat oven. Cut avocados in half and remove seed. If the seed is small you may need to scoop out extra meat to make room for the eggs. Sprinkle with any seasoning you like, crak one egg each avocado cup, bake until egg is cooked.

VARIATIONS/SUGGESTIONS:

- Serve with grapefruit or fruit of choice
- Serve with veggies

BASIC NUTRITION AND KEY VITAMINS/MINERALS PER SERVING							
Calories	Carbs (g)	Net Carbs (g)	Sugar (g)	Protein (g)	Fiber (g)	Fat (g)	Vitamins/Mineral
298	9	3	1	14	6	24	E, K, Copper,

FLAX FLATBREAD

Prep Time	15 Minutes
Cook /Chill Time	25-30 Minutes
Cook Temp (F)	350
Servings	12 Slices
Storage	Refrigerate
Storage Duration	10 Days

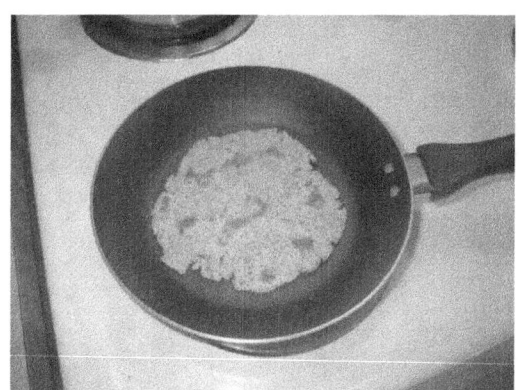

INGREDIENTS:

2 cups Ground Flax
½ cup Thai Kitchen Lite Coconut Milk
5 Tbsp Chia Seeds
1 cup Water
1 Tbsp Baking Soda

INSTRUCTIONS:

Preheat oven. Combine Chia Seeds and water, set aside to form egg substitute gel (10 minutes). Once the gell has formed combine all the ingredients in a large bowl, mixing well. Spred mixture evenly in a small rectangular pan (8X11-ish). Bake until edges start to crisp. Cut into 12 small square pieces/

VARIATIONS/SUGGESTIONS:

- Add spices prior to baking for a more flavorful bread
- Sub almond or coconut flour for flax if you prefer

BASIC NUTRITION AND KEY VITAMINS/MINERALS PER SERVING							
Calories	Carbs (g)	Net Carbs (g)	Sugar (g)	Protein (g)	Fiber (g)	Fat (g)	Vitamins/Mineral
111	9	2	0	5	7	6	Bs, C, D, E, Calcium

FOURTH OF JULY CHIA PARFAITS

Prep Time	10 Minutes
Cook /Chill Time	2 Hours/Overnight
Cook Temp (F)	NA
Servings	4
Storage	Refrigerate
Storage Duration	3 Days

INGREDIENTS:

Pudding:

    2 cups Unsweetened Almond Milk
    1 scoop Yoli Yes Shake Vanilla
    2/3 cup Chia Seed

Fruits:

    1 cup Fresh Blueberries
    1 cup Fresh Raspberried
    2 Tbsp Goji Berries

INSTRUCTIONS:

Make chia pudding and let chill/form up. In 4 cups, layer ¼ cup blueberries, ¼ cup of pudding, ¼ cup raspberries, remaining chia pudding, sprinkle with goji berries.

VARIATIONS/SUGGESTIONS:

- Add coconut, strawberries, nuts, seeds

BASIC NUTRITION AND KEY VITAMINS/MINERALS PER SERVING							
Calories	Carbs (g)	Net Carbs (g)	Sugar (g)	Protein (g)	Fiber (g)	Fat (g)	Vitamins/Mineral
280	23	13	13	12	10	12	D, E, Magnesium

GUACAMOLE

Prep Time	10 Minutes
Cook /Chill Time	NA
Cook Temp (F)	NA
Servings	2-4
Storage	Refrigerate
Storage Duration	4 Days

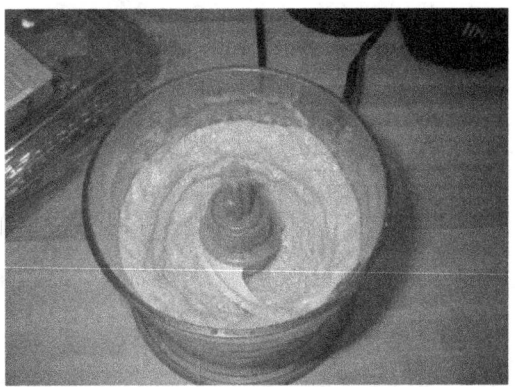

INGREDIENTS:

1 Avocado
1 large chopped Onion
1 chopped Roma Tomato
Juice of 1 Lemon
Juice of 1 Lime
2 tsp Cumin
1 tsp Black Pepper

INSTRUCTIONS:

Combine avocado, juices, cumin and pepper in a food processor until smooth. Pulse in tomato and onion.

VARIATIONS/SUGGESTIONS:

- For added spice, blend in jalapeno and cayenne pepper
- Nutrition based on 4 servings

BASIC NUTRITION AND KEY VITAMINS/MINERALS PER SERVING							
Calories	Carbs (g)	Net Carbs (g)	Sugar (g)	Protein (g)	Fiber (g)	Fat (g)	Vitamins/Mineral
42	8	6	3	1	2	5	C, E, K, Potassium

LEMON PIE CHIA PUDDING

Prep Time	5 Minutes
Cook /Chill Time	2 Hours/Overnight
Cook Temp (F)	NA
Servings	2
Storage	Refrigerate
Storage Duration	2 Days

INGREDIENTS:

Pudding:

> 2 peeled Lemons
> 1 cup Unsweetened Almond Milk
> 1 scoop Yoli Yes Shake Vanilla
> ¼ cup Chia Seed

Garnish (crust):

> 1 tsp Ginger
> 1 tsp Cinnamon
> 1 Tbsp Almonds

INSTRUCTIONS:

In a blender, pulse together garnish ingredients and set aside. In the same blender, combine the pudding ingredients, blending really well to ensure lemons get liquified. Pour into 2 cups, garnish, and chill.

VARIATIONS/SUGGESTIONS:

- Top with whipped coconut cream for a dessery treat

BASIC NUTRITION AND KEY VITAMINS/MINERALS PER SERVING							
Calories	Carbs (g)	Net Carbs (g)	Sugar (g)	Protein (g)	Fiber (g)	Fat (g)	Vitamins/Mineral
256	12	4	3	14	8	15	Mangonese, Zinc, Iron

LIME PIE CHIA PUDDING

Prep Time	5 Minutes
Cook /Chill Time	2 Hours/Overnight
Cook Temp (F)	NA
Servings	2
Storage	Refrigerate
Storage Duration	2 Days

INGREDIENTS:

Pudding:

    2 peeled Limes
    1 cup Unsweetened Almond Milk
    1 scoop Yoli Yes Shake Vanilla
    ¼ cup Chia Seed

Crust:

    2 Tbsp Coconut Oil
    1 tsp Ginger
    1 tsp Cinnamon
    1 Tbsp Almonds

INSTRUCTIONS:

In a blender, pulse together garnish ingredients and pour into two cups. In the same blender, combine the pudding ingredients, blending really well to ensure limes get liquified. Pour into cups and chill.

VARIATIONS/SUGGESTIONS:

- Top with whipped coconut cream for a dessery treat
- Use key limes to make it really yummy

BASIC NUTRITION AND KEY VITAMINS/MINERALS PER SERVING							
Calories	Carbs (g)	Net Carbs (g)	Sugar (g)	Protein (g)	Fiber (g)	Fat (g)	Vitamins/Mineral
437	18	7	3	16	11	33	Bs, C, Magnesium

Lox "Rice" Bowl

Prep Time	10 Minutes
Cook /Chill Time	20 Minutes
Cook Temp (F)	Medium
Servings	2
Storage	Refrigerate
Storage Duration	2 Days

INGREDIENTS:

2 cup Cauliflower Rice

1 cup finely chopped Baby Greens Mix
½ cup chopped Red Cabbage

1 Tbsp Avocado Oil
½ cup chopped Celery
1 medium diced Zucchini
1 medium chopped Carrot
6 chopped Asparagus Spears
9 halved Brussel Sprouts
½ cup chopped Snow Peas
½ lb diced Wild SalmonFillets
1 tsp Garlic Powder
1 tsp Sage

2 Tbsp Lemon Juice
1 Tbsp Dill

INSTRUCTIONS:

Make cauliflower rice. In a large skillet on medium heat, combine all ingredients from avocado oil to sage. Saute for about 20 minutes, or until salmon is to desired doneness. In two bowl, layer rice, greens and cabbage, and lox mix. Top with lemon juice and dill.

VARIATIONS/SUGGESTIONS:

- If you prefer smoked salmon, just saute the veggies and top with smoked salmon

BASIC NUTRITION AND KEY VITAMINS/MINERALS PER SERVING							
Calories	Carbs (g)	Net Carbs (g)	Sugar (g)	Protein (g)	Fiber (g)	Fat (g)	Vitamins/Mineral
440	28	17	9	41	11	20	C, Potassium, Iron

Mexican Mocha Protein Bowl

Prep Time	5 Minutes
Cook /Chill Time	Overnight
Cook Temp (F)	NA
Servings	2
Storage	Refrigerate
Storage Duration	2 Days

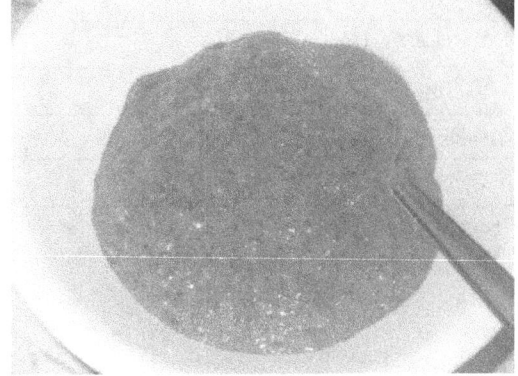

INGREDIENTS:

1 cup Unsweetened Almond Milk
½ cup Chia Seeds
¼ cup Coffee or Herbal Coffee Alternative
1 scoop Yoli Yes Shake Chocolate
2 tsp Cinnamon
2 tsp Chili Pepper
1 tsp Cayenne Pepper

INSTRUCTIONS:

Mix all ingredients and chill overnight.

VARIATIONS/SUGGESTIONS:

- As with all recipes, feel free to use your favorite protein powder or chocolate powder

BASIC NUTRITION AND KEY VITAMINS/MINERALS PER SERVING							
Calories	Carbs (g)	Net Carbs (g)	Sugar (g)	Protein (g)	Fiber (g)	Fat (g)	Vitamins/Mineral
193	19	4	1	13	15	8	Bs, E, Copper, Iron

No Mayo Chicken Salad

Prep Time	10 Minutes
Cook /Chill Time	NA
Cook Temp (F)	NA
Servings	4
Storage	Refrigerate
Storage Duration	4 Days

Ingredients:

2 cups diced cooked Chicken
1 medium Apple of choice (or 1 cup variety mix)
¼ cup diced Red Onion
¼ cup diced Zucchini
¼ cup diced Cucumber
3 Tbsp Tahini
1 Tbsp Sunflower Seeds
1 Tbsp chopped Walnuts
1 Tbsp sliced Almonds
1 Tbsp Avocado Oil

Instructions:

Whisk together tahini and avocado oil. In a separate bowl combine the rest of the ingredients, pour tahini dresing over the top, and mix together well.

Variations/Suggestions:

- Great on veggie chips or in lettuce wraps

Basic Nutrition and Key Vitamins/Minerals Per Serving							
Calories	Carbs (g)	Net Carbs (g)	Sugar (g)	Protein (g)	Fiber (g)	Fat (g)	Vitamins/Mineral
280	8	6	5	26	2	19	C, E, Copper

NO MAYO EGG SALAD

Prep Time	5 Minutes
Cook /Chill Time	NA
Cook Temp (F)	NA
Servings	2
Storage	Refrigerate
Storage Duration	4 Days

INGREDIENTS:

4 hard boiled Eggs
1 Avocado
¼ cup diced Red Onion
¼ cup diced Celery
2 tsp Lemon Juice
1 tsp Lime Juice
1 tsp Sririacha

INSTRUCTIONS:

Combine the avocado, lemon juice, and sriracha in a food processor until smooth. Pulse in the onion and celery. Cut the eggs into four parts and pulse or mix in with a fork.

VARIATIONS/SUGGESTIONS:

- Great for lettuce wraps or on sunflower bread
- Garnish with tomato, sprouts, carrots, etc.

BASIC NUTRITION AND KEY VITAMINS/MINERALS PER SERVING							
Calories	Carbs (g)	Net Carbs (g)	Sugar (g)	Protein (g)	Fiber (g)	Fat (g)	Vitamins/Mineral
288	6	1	2	15	5	22	C, E, K, Copper

PECAN PIE CHIA PUDDING

Prep Time	5 Minutes
Cook /Chill Time	15 Min / 2 Hours
Cook Temp (F)	Medium-Low
Servings	2
Storage	Refrigerate
Storage Duration	2 Days

INGREDIENTS:

Pudding:

      1 cup Unsweetened Almond Milk
      1 scoop Yoli Yes Shake Vanilla
      3 Tbsp Chia Seeds
      2 tsp Cinnamon

Sauce:

      ½ cup Unsweetened Almond Milk
      2 pitted Medjool Dates
      ½ cup Pecan Pieces

INSTRUCTIONS:

Make pudding and chill. Before serving, in a saucepan bring the milk and dates to a low boil. Let simmer for 10 minutes. Transfer to a food processor, leaving the heat on the pan and adding the pecans into the pan. Pulse the milk and dates into a liquid, transfer back to pot, let simmer with pecans for 5 more minutes/ Spoon the mixture onto the chia pudding.

VARIATIONS/SUGGESTIONS:

- All ingredients can be made together and chilled
- Top with shredded coconut for extra flavor

BASIC NUTRITION AND KEY VITAMINS/MINERALS PER SERVING							
Calories	Carbs (g)	Net Carbs (g)	Sugar (g)	Protein (g)	Fiber (g)	Fat (g)	Vitamins/Mineral
414	37	23	18	13	14	28	E, Magnesium

PUMPKIN PIE CHIA PUDDING

Prep Time	5 Minutes
Cook /Chill Time	2 Hours
Cook Temp (F)	NA
Servings	2
Storage	Refrigerate
Storage Duration	2 Days

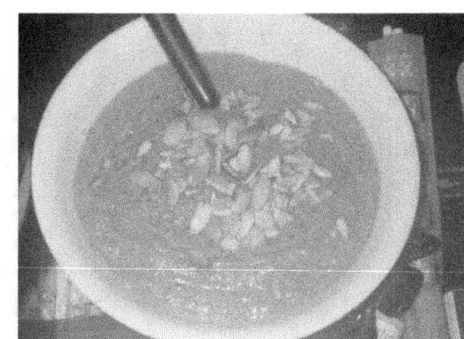

INGREDIENTS:

½ cup Pumpkin Puree
1/3 cup Thai Kitchen Lite Coconut Milk
1/3 cup Water
¼ cup Chia Seeds
2 tsp Cinnamon
2 tsp Allspice
1 tsp Ginger
½ tsp Clove

INSTRUCTIONS:

Blend together everything minus the chia seeds, ensuring spices don't clump. Stir in chia seeds and chill.

VARIATIONS/SUGGESTIONS:

- Top with whipped coconut cream for a healthy dessert
- Much healthier than traditional pumpkin pie

BASIC NUTRITION AND KEY VITAMINS/MINERALS PER SERVING							
Calories	Carbs (g)	Net Carbs (g)	Sugar (g)	Protein (g)	Fiber (g)	Fat (g)	Vitamins/Mineral
170	15	4	2	7	11	8	Bs, E, Phosphorus

SALMON BAKED AVOCADO

Prep Time	5 Minutes
Cook /Chill Time	10 -20 Minutes
Cook Temp (F)	425
Servings	2-4
Storage	Refrigerate
Storage Duration	1 Day

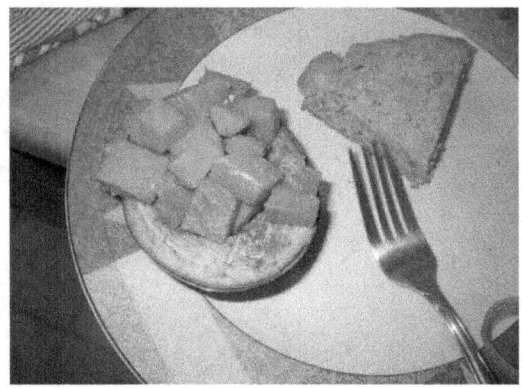

INGREDIENTS:

2 Avocado
8 oz raw cubed Salmon Fillet

INSTRUCTIONS:

Preheat oven. Slice open the avocado and remove the pit. Fill the avocado halves with the diced salmon and bake uncovered for 10-20 minutes, depending on how done you want the salmon.

VARIATIONS/SUGGESTIONS:

- Sprinkle with seasoning of chioce prior to baking (lemon juice and dill are good)
- Top with sriracha for a spicy kick

BASIC NUTRITION AND KEY VITAMINS/MINERALS PER SERVING							
Calories	Carbs (g)	Net Carbs (g)	Sugar (g)	Protein (g)	Fiber (g)	Fat (g)	Vitamins/Mineral
303	8	2	0	23	6	21	C, K, Copper, Iron

SHRIMP AND GARLIC BAKED AVOCADO

Prep Time	10 Minutes
Cook /Chill Time	30 Minutes
Cook Temp (F)	350
Servings	2
Storage	Refrigerate
Storage Duration	2 Days

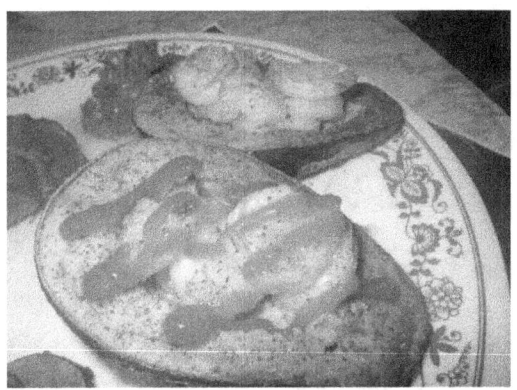

INGREDIENTS:

    20 medium-small Shrimp
    2 Avocado
    2 Tbsp minced Garlic
    1 tsp Chili Powder
    1 tsp Black Pepper

INSTRUCTIONS:

Preheat oven. Cut avocados in half and remove the seed. Sprinkle with chili powder and pepper. In a small saucepan on medium-low heat saute the shrimp and garlic for about 5 minutes, not quite cooking it all the way. Spoon shrimp into the avocado halves, cover, and bake for 20 minutes.

VARIATIONS/SUGGESTIONS:

- Serve with sauted veggies
- Top with sriracha for extra zing

BASIC NUTRITION AND KEY VITAMINS/MINERALS PER SERVING							
Calories	Carbs (g)	Net Carbs (g)	Sugar (g)	Protein (g)	Fiber (g)	Fat (g)	Vitamins/Mineral
272	16	6	1	12	1o	20	C, K, Calcium, Zinc

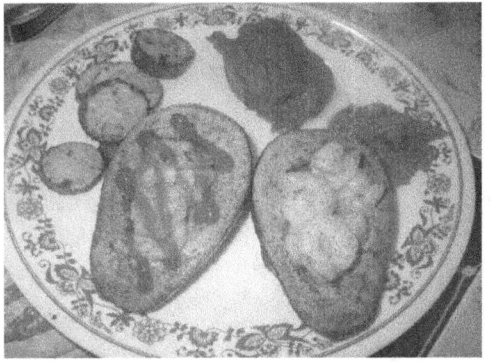

SPICY SALMON ATOP SPAGHETTI SQUASH

Prep Time	5 Minutes
Cook /Chill Time	1 hour 20 Minutes
Cook Temp (F)	375 / Medium High
Servings	4
Storage	Refrigerate
Storage Duration	3 Days

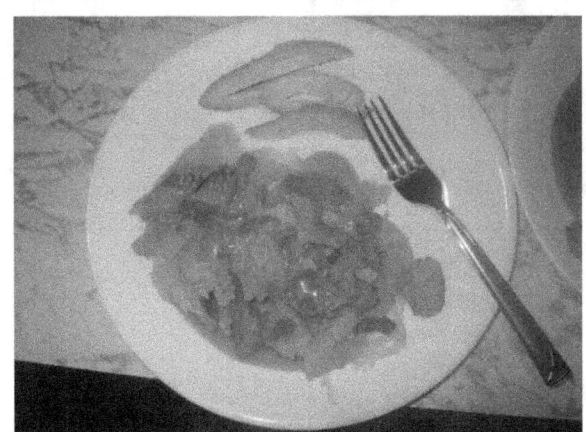

INGREDIENTS:

1 Spaghetti Squash, cut in half, seeds removed
1 lb cubed Salmon Fillet
1 cup Thai Kitchen Coconut Milk Lite
1 Tbsp minced Garlic
¼ cup Sriracha
1 ½ cup diced Capsicum
1 sliced Avocado

INSTRUCTIONS:

Preheat oven. Sprinkle the spaghetti squash with water and bake cut side down for 45 minutes-1 hour. In a medium saucepan, combine all the ingredients minus the capsicum and avocado. Cover and cook on medium heat for about 20 minutes (don't let the salmon dry out). Using a fork, remove the spaghetti squash from its skin. Layer spaghetti squash, capsicum, spicy salmon, and garnish with avocado.

VARIATIONS/SUGGESTIONS:

- Top with seaweed chips or sesame seeds for extra flavor
- If the salmon is good quality, leave it raw and don't heat the sauce

BASIC NUTRITION AND KEY VITAMINS/MINERALS PER SERVING							
Calories	Carbs (g)	Net Carbs (g)	Sugar (g)	Protein (g)	Fiber (g)	Fat (g)	Vitamins/Mineral
409	25	19	11	28	6	21	C, K, Calcium, Sodium

SUNFLOWER SODA BREAD

Prep Time	10 Minutes
Cook /Chill Time	45 Minutes
Cook Temp (F)	425
Servings	8-16
Storage	Refrigerate/Freeze
Storage Duration	5 Days/1 Month

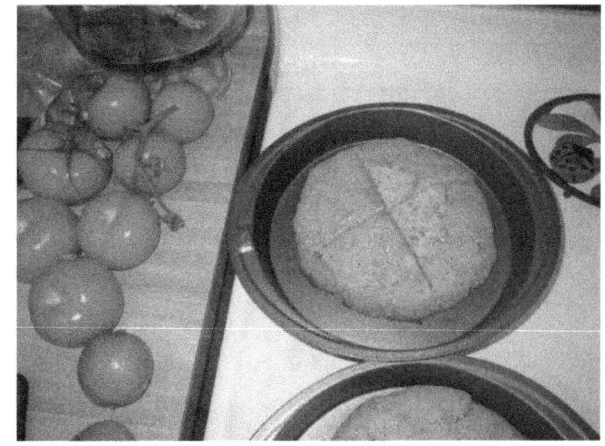

INGREDIENTS:

2 cup Almond Flour
1 ½ cup Coconut Flour
½ cup Flax/Chia Blend
1 ½ tsp Baking Soda
½ cup Sunflower Seeds
½ pureed Grapefruit (should yeild 1 cup)
1 can Thai Kitchen Coconut Milk Lite

INSTRUCTIONS:

Preheat oven. Combine dry ingredients in a bowl, slowly stir in grapefruit and milk. Knead until the dough holds together and has no clumps. Split into two balls and place them on a lined/oiled cookie sheet. Lightly cut an X on each top, cover, and bake for 30 minutes. Remove covering and bake 15 minutes, or until it reaches a nice brown color.

VARIATIONS/SUGGESTIONS:

- Sunflower seeds will turn green, they are still safe to eat
- Store in fridge as it will mold quicker than traditional breads
- Nutrition is based on 8 servings

BASIC NUTRITION AND KEY VITAMINS/MINERALS PER SERVING							
Calories	Carbs (g)	Net Carbs (g)	Sugar (g)	Protein (g)	Fiber (g)	Fat (g)	Vitamins/Mineral
338	26	19	2	9	7	23	Bs, C, E, Selenium

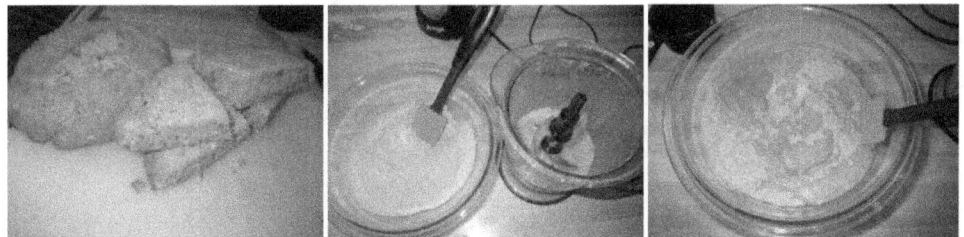

TUNA BRUSCHETTA PATTIES

Prep Time	5 Minutes
Cook /Chill Time	10-15 Min / 20 Min.
Cook Temp (F)	350
Servings	6
Storage	Refrigerate
Storage Duration	6 Days

INGREDIENTS:

1 cup cooked Tuna
½ cup diced Red Onion
¼ cup minced Garlic
1 Egg
2 quartered Roma Tomato
1 Tbsp Fresh Basil
1 Tbsp Flax
1 tsp Avocado Oil

INSTRUCTIONS:

Combine all ingredients in a food procesor and blend well. Chill for 20 minutes. Preheat oven and line or oil a cookie sheet. Form paste into 6 patties. Bake 10-15 minutes, until firm.

VARIATIONS/SUGGESTIONS:

- Serve in lettuce wraps with avocado and cucumber

BASIC NUTRITION AND KEY VITAMINS/MINERALS PER SERVING							
Calories	Carbs (g)	Net Carbs (g)	Sugar (g)	Protein (g)	Fiber (g)	Fat (g)	Vitamins/Mineral
113	8	7	2	8	1	6	C, K, Potassium

VANILLA PROTEIN FLAX CEREAL

Prep Time	10 Minutes
Cook /Chill Time	15-20 Minutes
Cook Temp (F)	350
Servings	8
Storage	Air Tight Container
Storage Duration	1 Month

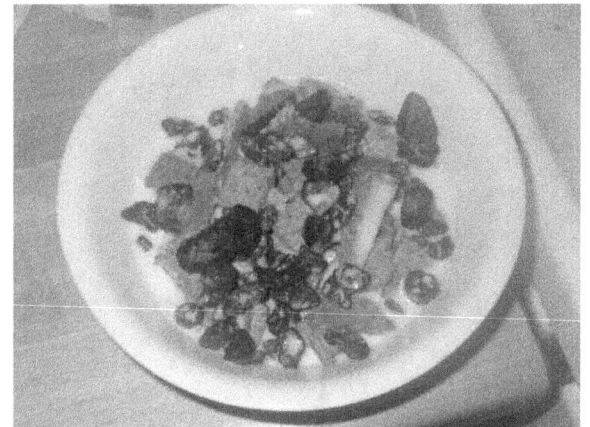

INGREDIENTS:

2 ½ cup Almond Flour
1 ¼ cup Flax
1 scoop Yoli Yes Shake Vanilla
1 Tbsp Cinnamon
½ cup Unsweetened Almond Milk
2 Tbsp Avocado/Coconut Oil Blend
2 Egg

INSTRUCTIONS:

Pulse ingredients together in a blender. Roll out between parchment paper to roughly an 1/8 inch thickness. Place bootom parchment paper on a cookie sheet, score lightly with a knife, and bake fo 15-20 minutes (should be deep golden but not burned). Let cool for 30 minutes and then break apart.

VARIATIONS/SUGGESTIONS:

- Add dried fruit to jazz it up
- Break into tiny pieces and mix with nuts/seeds for a grain free granola

BASIC NUTRITION AND KEY VITAMINS/MINERALS PER SERVING							
Calories	Carbs (g)	Net Carbs (g)	Sugar (g)	Protein (g)	Fiber (g)	Fat (g)	Vitamins/Mineral
245	13	4	0	13	0	25	Copper, Selenium

Natural Sweets

Almond Butter Oatmeal Squares

Almond Butter "Rice" Pudding

Apple Snack Squares

Apple Butter "Rice" Pudding

Banana Nut Oatcakes

Banana Oat Cookies

Black Bean Mocha Muffins

Chocolate Protein Pancakes

Cinnamon Pumpkin Cookies

Cinnamon Roll Nut Butter

Coconut "Rice" Pudding

"Cookie Dough" Bites

No Flour Pancakes

Pumpkin Almond Butter Bites

Pumpkin No Bake Cookies

Pumpkin "Rice" Pudding

Slow Cooker Berry Crisp

Triple Berry Nut Pies (Mock Cheesecake)

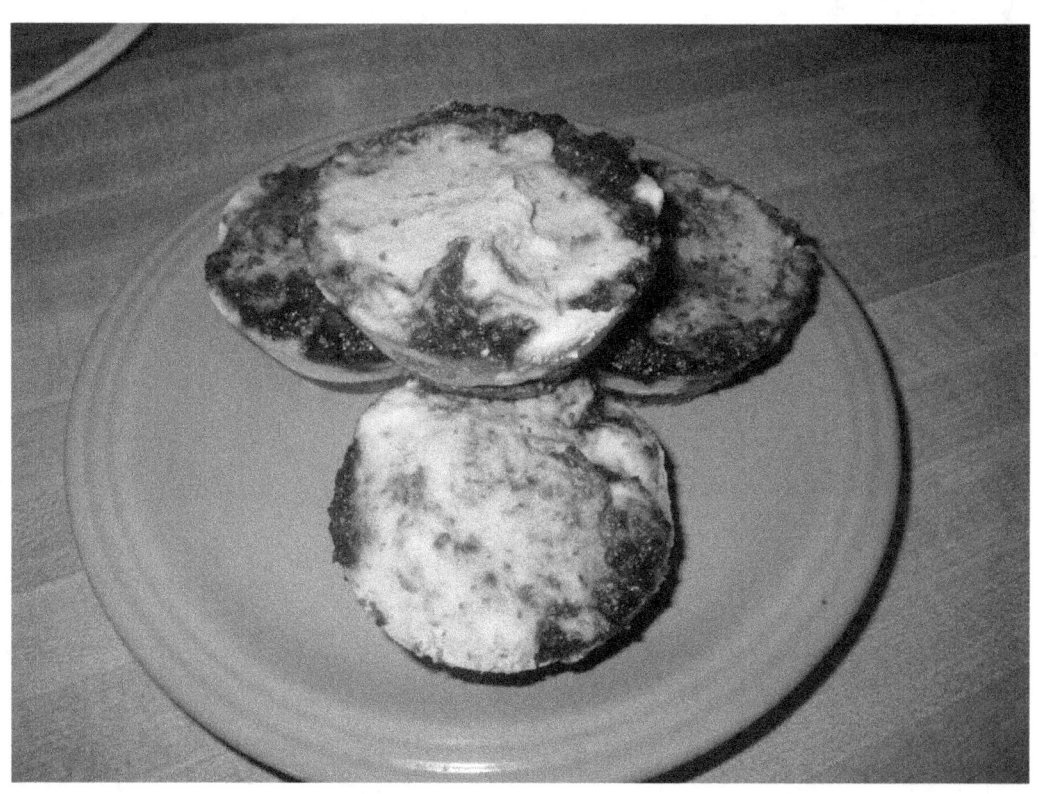

ALMOND BUTTER OATMEAL SQUARES

Prep Time	5 Minutes
Cook /Chill Time	20-30 Minutes
Cook Temp (F)	350
Servings	9
Storage	Refrigerate
Storage Duration	1 Week

INGREDIENTS:

3 scoop Yoli Yes Shake Vanilla
2 cup Unsweetened Almond Milk
1 cup Low Sodium Chickpeas
1 cup Steele Cut Oats
¼ cup Almond Butter
3 Tbsp Coconut Oil
2 tsp Cinnamon
1 tsp Baking Soda
½ tsp Nutmeg
1 Egg

INSTRUCTIONS:

Preheat oven. Combine all ingredients in a blender. Pour inot greased 9X9 pan. Bake for 25-30 minutes, let sit 10 minutes before cutting into squares.

VARIATIONS/SUGGESTIONS:

- Add dark choclate chips or chocolate protein powder for a yummy kick
- Use 2 ripe bananas instead of egg if you like

BASIC NUTRITION AND KEY VITAMINS/MINERALS PER SERVING							
Calories	Carbs (g)	Net Carbs (g)	Sugar (g)	Protein (g)	Fiber (g)	Fat (g)	Vitamins/Mineral
185	16	11	1	9	5	10	C, E, Magnesium

ALMOND BUTTER "RICE" PUDDING

Prep Time	5 Minutes
Cook /Chill Time	20 Minutes
Cook Temp (F)	Medium Low
Servings	2
Storage	Refrigerate
Storage Duration	2 Days

INGREDIENTS:

    1 ½ cup Cauliflower Rice
    1 cup Usweetened Almond Milk
    2 Tbsp Almond Butter
    1 ripe Banana
    1 tsp Cinnamon

INSTRUCTIONS:

In a blender, blend all ingredients except the cauliflower rice to a smooth consistency. In a saucepan, bring the mixture and the rice to a boil, then simmer for 15-20 minutes.

VARIATIONS/SUGGESTIONS:

- Garnish with extra cinnamon/spice
- Add vanilla protein powder for extra sweetness/protein boost

BASIC NUTRITION AND KEY VITAMINS/MINERALS PER SERVING							
Calories	Carbs (g)	Net Carbs (g)	Sugar (g)	Protein (g)	Fiber (g)	Fat (g)	Vitamins/Mineral
198	23	17	12	5	6	12	Manganese, Iron, Zinc

APPLE SNACK SQUARES

Prep Time	10 Minutes
Cook /Chill Time	1 Hour
Cook Temp (F)	375
Servings	9
Storage	Refrigerate
Storage Duration	4 Days

INGREDIENTS:

2 cup Cauliflower Rice
2 medium diced Apples
2 Eggs
2 cup Unsweetened Almond Milk
½ cup No Sugar Added Raisins
1/3 cup chopped Almonds
1 scoop Yoli Yes Shake Vanilla
2 tsp Cinnamon
1 tsp Nutmeg
½ tsp Ginger

INSTRUCTIONS:

Preheat oven and oil a 9X9 baking pan. Layer riced cauliflower, diced apples, raisins, spices, and almonds. Whip eggs, vanilla powder and milk together and pour over mixture. Bake covered for 1 hour. Let stand 5 minutes prior to serving.

VARIATIONS/SUGGESTIONS:

- Add almond or coconut meal for a cookie-like bar

BASIC NUTRITION AND KEY VITAMINS/MINERALS PER SERVING							
Calories	Carbs (g)	Net Carbs (g)	Sugar (g)	Protein (g)	Fiber (g)	Fat (g)	Vitamins/Mineral
95	12	9	7	4	3	4	C, E, Magnesium

APPLE BUTTER "RICE" PUDDING

Prep Time	5 Minutes
Cook /Chill Time	20 Minutes
Cook Temp (F)	Low
Servings	2
Storage	Refrigerate
Storage Duration	2 Days

INGREDIENTS:

1 ½ cup Cauliflower Rice
1 cup Unsweetened Almond Milk
1 cup Unsweetened Apple Butter or Sauce
1 tsp Cinnamon

INSTRUCTIONS:

In a saucepan, combine all ingredients and bring to boil. Reduce and simmer 20 minutes.

VARIATIONS/SUGGESTIONS:

- Add vanilla protein powder for a protein kick

BASIC NUTRITION AND KEY VITAMINS/MINERALS PER SERVING							
Calories	Carbs (g)	Net Carbs (g)	Sugar (g)	Protein (g)	Fiber (g)	Fat (g)	Vitamins/Mineral
280	65	60	52	3	5	2	A, C, E, Copper

BANANA NUT PROTEIN OATCAKES

Prep Time	5 Minutes
Cook /Chill Time	10 Minutes
Cook Temp (F)	Medium High
Servings	2
Storage	Refrigerate
Storage Duration	2 Days

INGREDIENTS:

2 Banana
1 cup Steele Cut Oats
1 cup Unsweetened Almond Milk
1 scoop Yoli Yes Shake Vanilla
2 tsp Cinnamon
1 Tsp Baking Soda

INSTRUCTIONS:

In a blender, combine all ingredients. In a heated, lightly oiled pan, pour batter into 4 inch cakes. Once the edges buble, flip and cook until golden (about 4 minutes).

VARIATIONS/SUGGESTIONS:

- Top with almond butter
- Add fruits/nuts

BASIC NUTRITION AND KEY VITAMINS/MINERALS PER SERVING							
Calories	Carbs (g)	Net Carbs (g)	Sugar (g)	Protein (g)	Fiber (g)	Fat (g)	Vitamins/Mineral
266	44	37	9	12	7	2	Bs, E, Magnesium

BANANA OAT COOKIES

Prep Time	10 Minutes
Cook /Chill Time	10-15 Minutes
Cook Temp (F)	350
Servings	4
Storage	Air Tight Container
Storage Duration	1 Week

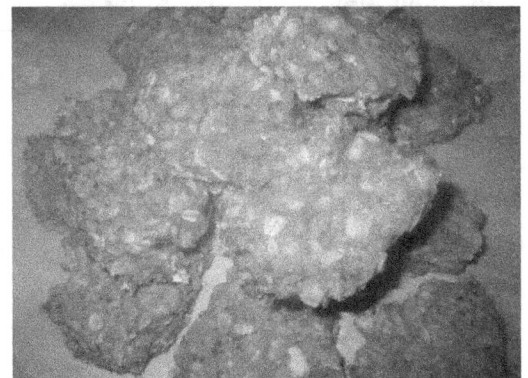

INGREDIENTS:

2 Banana
1 cup Steele Cut Oats
1 Tbsp Almond Butter
2 tsp Chia
2 tsp Flax
2 tsp Cinnamon

INSTRUCTIONS:

Combine all ingredients in a blender and let sit for 10 minutes. Preheat oven. On a lined or oiled cookie sheet, form four cookies. Bake 10-15 minutes (too dry and they will crumble apart).

VARIATIONS/SUGGESTIONS:

- If they come out to crumbly, mix with nuts/seeds for granola
- Use any nut/seed butter you like

BASIC NUTRITION AND KEY VITAMINS/MINERALS PER SERVING							
Calories	Carbs (g)	Net Carbs (g)	Sugar (g)	Protein (g)	Fiber (g)	Fat (g)	Vitamins/Mineral
170	27	21	6	4	6	3	Potassium, Copper

Black Bean Mocha Muffins

Prep Time	10 Minutes
Cook /Chill Time	15-20 Minutes
Cook Temp (F)	350
Servings	10
Storage	Refrigerate/Freeze
Storage Duration	5 Days/2 Months

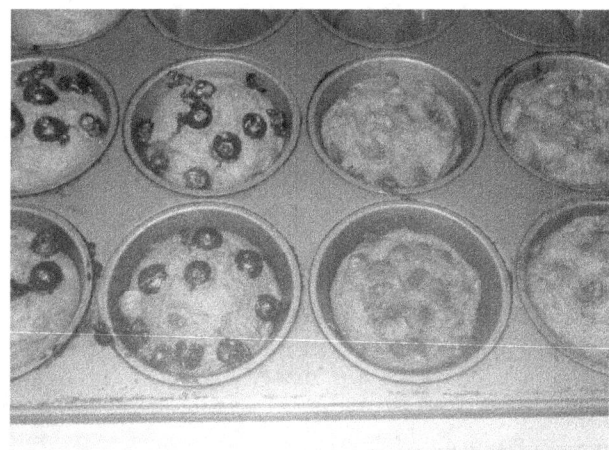

INGREDIENTS:

1 cup Low Sodium Black Beans
1 cup Almond Butter
2 scoops Yoli Yes Shake Chocolate
2 Tbsp Flax
5 Tbsp Coffee or Coffee Alternative
1 Tbsp Avocado/Coconut Oil Blend
1 Tbsp Cinnamon
1 tsp Baking Soda

INSTRUCTIONS:

Combine flax and coffee in abowl and set aside. Preheat oven. Rinse and drain beans. In a blender or food processor, combine beansand almond butter into a paste. Add the rest of the ingredients including the flax/coffe mix and blend. Spoon batter into an oil/lined muffin tin, filling the cups 2/3 of the way.

VARIATIONS/SUGGESTIONS:

- Top with nuts/seeds
- "Frost" with good quality chocolate nutbutter (NOT Nutella)

BASIC NUTRITION AND KEY VITAMINS/MINERALS PER SERVING							
Calories	Carbs (g)	Net Carbs (g)	Sugar (g)	Protein (g)	Fiber (g)	Fat (g)	Vitamins/Mineral
218	11	5	1	9	6	17	Bs, C, E, Sodium

Chocolate Protein Pancakes

Prep Time	5 Minutes
Cook /Chill Time	10 Minutes
Cook Temp (F)	Medium High
Servings	2
Storage	Refrigerate
Storage Duration	2 Days

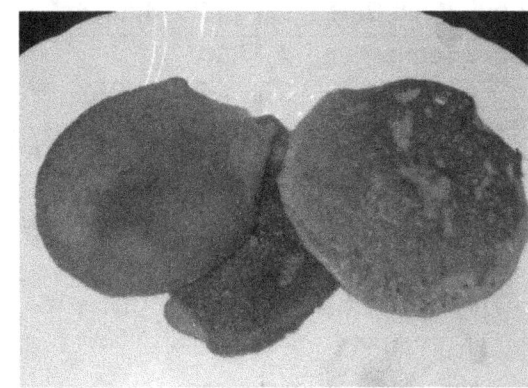

INGREDIENTS:

- 1 ½ cup Unsweetened Almond Milk
- 2 scoop Yoli Yes Shake Chocolate
- 2 Egg
- 2 tsp Red Pepper
- 1 tsp Baking Soda

INSTRUCTIONS:

In a blender, combine all ingredients. In a heated/oiled pan, pour batter into 4 inch cakes. Once the edges have bubbled, flip and cook until done (about 4 minutes).

VARIATIONS/SUGGESTIONS:

- Ma

BASIC NUTRITION AND KEY VITAMINS/MINERALS PER SERVING							
Calories	Carbs (g)	Net Carbs (g)	Sugar (g)	Protein (g)	Fiber (g)	Fat (g)	Vitamins/Mineral
190	10	5	2	19	5	9	Bs, E, Magnesium

Cinnamon Pumpkin Cookies

Prep Time	5 Minutes
Cook /Chill Time	10-15 Minutes
Cook Temp (F)	350
Servings	12
Storage	Air Tight Container
Storage Duration	10 Days

Ingredients:

1 cup Almond Flour
1 cup Coconut Flour
½ cup Pumpkin Puree
3 Tbsp softened Coconut Oil
2 scoop Yoli Yes Shake Vanilla
1 Tbsp Cinnamon
½ tsp Baking Soda

Instructions:

Preheat oven. Mix dry and wet ingredients in separate bowls. Slowly mix wet and dry together, mixing well. Roll into 12 balls, place on lined/oiled cookie sheet and squash to desired thickness. Bake to golden brown.

Variations/Suggestions:

- Dust with cinnamon/palm sugar mix for extra sweetness

BASIC NUTRITION AND KEY VITAMINS/MINERALS PER SERVING							
Calories	Carbs (g)	Net Carbs (g)	Sugar (g)	Protein (g)	Fiber (g)	Fat (g)	Vitamins/Mineral
144	10	4	5	5	6	10	A, C, E, Selenium

CINNAMON ROLL NUT BUTTER

Prep Time	5 Minutes
Cook /Chill Time	Overnight
Cook Temp (F)	NA
Servings	16
Storage	Refrigerate
Storage Duration	3 Weeks

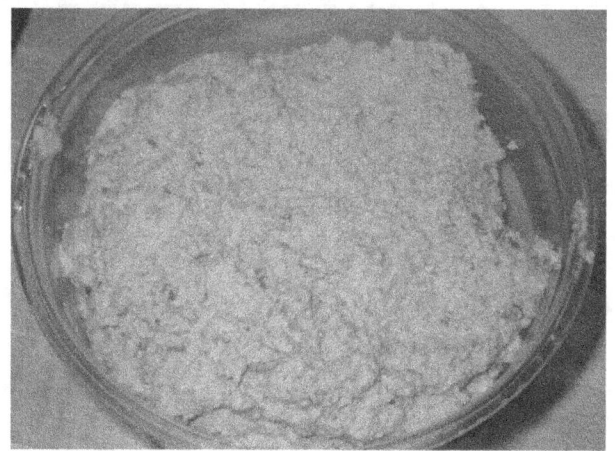

INGREDIENTS:

1 scoop Yoli Yes Shake Vanilla
1 cup Almonds
¾ cup Walnuts
4 Pitted Medjool Dates
3 Tbsp Almond/Coconut Oil Blend
3 Tbsp Unsweetened Almond Milk
2 Tbsp Cinnamon

INSTRUCTIONS:

Soak the nuts and dates in water overnight to soften. Drain and blend all ingredients in a blender until smooth.

VARIATIONS/SUGGESTIONS:

- Really yummy spread on apples
- Anti Inflammatory

BASIC NUTRITION AND KEY VITAMINS/MINERALS PER SERVING							
Calories	Carbs (g)	Net Carbs (g)	Sugar (g)	Protein (g)	Fiber (g)	Fat (g)	Vitamins/Mineral
126	8	6	5	3	2	10	Potassium, Copper

COCONUT "RICE" PUDDING

Prep Time	5 Minutes
Cook /Chill Time	20 Minutes
Cook Temp (F)	Low
Servings	2
Storage	Refrigerate
Storage Duration	2 Days

INGREDIENTS:

1 ½ cup Culiflower Rice
1 cup Unsweetened Coconut Milk
1 Banana
1 scoop Yoli Yes Shake Vanilla
1 Tbsp Coconut Oil

INSTRUCTIONS:

Blend all ingredients, minus the cauliflower, together in a food processor or blender. Combine all ingredients in a saucepan, bring to boil and then reduce to simmer.

VARIATIONS/SUGGESTIONS:

- Top with spice/fruit/nuts for added flavor

BASIC NUTRITION AND KEY VITAMINS/MINERALS PER SERVING							
Calories	Carbs (g)	Net Carbs (g)	Sugar (g)	Protein (g)	Fiber (g)	Fat (g)	Vitamins/Mineral
197	24	18	12	8	6	10	Bs, C, E, Potassium

"COOKIE DOUGH" PROTEIN BITES

Prep Time	10 Minutes
Cook /Chill Time	NA
Cook Temp (F)	NA
Servings	6
Storage	Refrigerate
Storage Duration	6 Days

INGREDIENTS:

1 ½ cup Unsweetened Coconut Flakes
2/3 cup dried No Sugar Added Fruit Medley (dates, figs etc.)
1 scoop Yoli Yes Shake Vanilla
2 tsp Cinnamon
1 tsp Flax
1 tsp Nutmeg

INSTRUCTIONS:

Combine all ingredients in a blender and blend well. Roll into bite sized balls and enjoy.

VARIATIONS/SUGGESTIONS:

- Add coconut oil if the mix is too dry
- Roll in cacao powder for a chocolate fix

BASIC NUTRITION AND KEY VITAMINS/MINERALS PER SERVING							
Calories	Carbs (g)	Net Carbs (g)	Sugar (g)	Protein (g)	Fiber (g)	Fat (g)	Vitamins/Mineral
130	12	8	5	9	4	8	Bs, C, E, Copper, Zinc

No Flour Cinn. Protein Pancakes

Prep Time	5 Minutes
Cook /Chill Time	10 Minutes
Cook Temp (F)	Medium High
Servings	2
Storage	Refrigerate
Storage Duration	2 Days

INGREDIENTS:

2 Banana
1 ½ cup Unsweetened Almond Milk
1 scoop Yoli Yes Shake Vanilla
1 Egg
2 tsp Cinnamon
1 tsp Baking Soda

INSTRUCTIONS:

Combine all ingredients in a blender. In a heated, lightly oiled pan, pour batter into 4 inch cakes. Once the edges have bubbled, flip and cook until brown (about 4 minutes).

VARIATIONS/SUGGESTIONS:

- Add raisins/ginger for added flavor

BASIC NUTRITION AND KEY VITAMINS/MINERALS PER SERVING							
Calories	Carbs (g)	Net Carbs (g)	Sugar (g)	Protein (g)	Fiber (g)	Fat (g)	Vitamins/Mineral
218	34	29	21	12	5	6	Bs, E, Manganese

PUMPKIN ALMOND BUTTER BITES

Prep Time	10 Minutes
Cook /Chill Time	NA
Cook Temp (F)	NA
Servings	30-40
Storage	Refrigerate/Counter
Storage Duration	10 Days

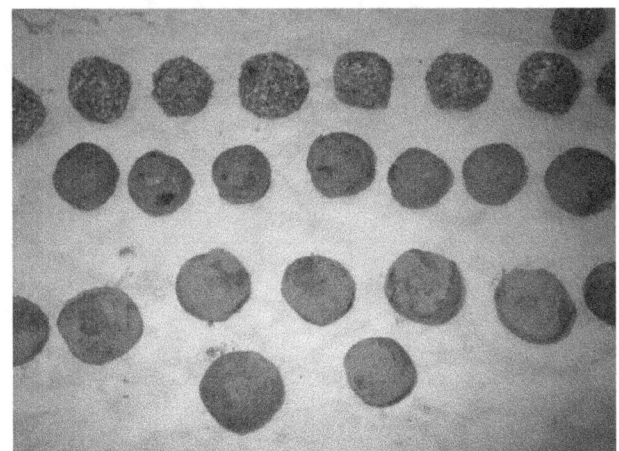

INGREDIENTS:

½ cup Pumkin Puree
½ cup Almond Butter
½ cup Coconut Flour
¼ cup Fig Spread
1 scoop Yoli Yes Shake Vanilla
1 Tbsp Cinnamon
1 tsp Nutmeg

INSTRUCTIONS:

Mix all ingredients together. Roll into bite size balls.

VARIATIONS/SUGGESTIONS:

- Add nuts/seeds for added crunch
- Nutrition is based on 30 servings

BASIC NUTRITION AND KEY VITAMINS/MINERALS PER SERVING							
Calories	Carbs (g)	Net Carbs (g)	Sugar (g)	Protein (g)	Fiber (g)	Fat (g)	Vitamins/Mineral
42	4	2	2	3	2	3	Magnesium, Copper

PUMPKIN NO BAKE COOKIES

Prep Time	10 Minutes
Cook /Chill Time	25 Minutes/2 Hours
Cook Temp (F)	Medium Low
Servings	16
Storage	Refrigerate/Counter
Storage Duration	7 Days

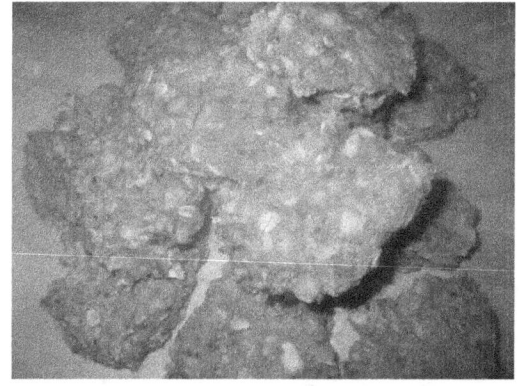

INGREDIENTS:

1 can Pumpkin Puree
1 1/3 cup Steele Cut Oats
1 cup Flax/Chia Blend
¾ cup Muesli
½ cup Coconut Flour
½ cup Thai Kitchen Lite Coconut Milk
12 pitted Medjool Dates
2 Tbsp Cinnamon
2 tsp Allspice
2 tsp Nutmeg
1 tsp Ginger

INSTRUCTIONS:

In a medium pot, simmer coconut milk and dates for 10 minutes. Pour milk and dates in food processor and blend until smooth, add pumpkin and mix well. Return to pan on low heat, add spices and let simmer for 15 minutes. Turn off the heat, add flours, oats, and muesli. Drop cookies onto wax paper and let sit for a few hours. Once they have cooled, store in an air tight container in the fridge or on the counter.

VARIATIONS/SUGGESTIONS:

- Add dried fruit bits if you like

BASIC NUTRITION AND KEY VITAMINS/MINERALS PER SERVING							
Calories	Carbs (g)	Net Carbs (g)	Sugar (g)	Protein (g)	Fiber (g)	Fat (g)	Vitamins/Mineral
130	26	20	15	4	6	4	Magnesium, Sodium

PUMPKIN "RICE" PUDDING

Prep Time	5 Minutes
Cook /Chill Time	20 Minutes
Cook Temp (F)	Low
Servings	2
Storage	Refrigerate
Storage Duration	2 Days

INGREDIENTS:

1 ½ cup Cauliflower Rice
1 cup Unsweetened Almond Milk
1 cup Pumpkin Puree
1 scoop Yoli Yes Shake Vanilla
2 tsp Allspice
1 tsp Cinnamon

INSTRUCTIONS:

Combine all ingredients in a saucepan. Bring to a boil, then cover and let simmer for 20 minutes.

VARIATIONS/SUGGESTIONS:

- Add almond butter for a crust like flavor
- Top with extra spice/nuts/seeds

BASIC NUTRITION AND KEY VITAMINS/MINERALS PER SERVING							
Calories	Carbs (g)	Net Carbs (g)	Sugar (g)	Protein (g)	Fiber (g)	Fat (g)	Vitamins/Mineral
133	19	12	8	9	7	2	Phosphorus, Copper

SLOW COOKER BERRY CRISP

Prep Time	5 Minutes
Cook /Chill Time	2-3 Hours
Cook Temp (F)	Low
Servings	4
Storage	Refrigerate
Storage Duration	3 Days

INGREDIENTS:

4 medium cored and diced Apples
1 cup raw Cranberries
1 cup raw Blueberries
½ cup Almond Flour
¼ cup Almonds
¼ cup Unsweetened Shredded Coconut
1 Tbsp Cinnamon
½ cup Water

INSTRUCTIONS:

In a blender, lightly pulse together the flour, cinnamon, almond and coconut. Layer fruit, ½ cup water, then mix in the slow cooker. Cook on low.

VARIATIONS/SUGGESTIONS:

- Add extra seeds/nuts for enhanced flavor

BASIC NUTRITION AND KEY VITAMINS/MINERALS PER SERVING							
Calories	Carbs (g)	Net Carbs (g)	Sugar (g)	Protein (g)	Fiber (g)	Fat (g)	Vitamins/Mineral
279	36	27	20	6	9	16	E, Selenium, Copper

TRIPLE BERRY NUT PIES

Prep Time	2 Hours
Cook /Chill Time	20 minutes/Overnight
Cook Temp (F)	Medium
Servings	12
Storage	Refrigerate/Freeze
Storage Duration	2 Days/1 Month

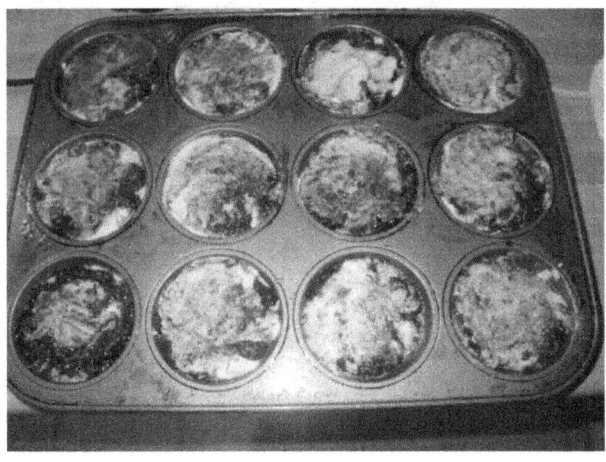

INGREDIENTS:

Crust:

    12 Pitted Medjool Dates
    ¼ cup Almonds
    ¼ cup Walnuts
    2 Tbsp Tahini
    2 tsp Cinnamon
    1 tsp Ginger
    1 tsp Allspice

Filling

    1 ¼ cup soaked Cahew/Almond/Macadamia Blend
    2 cup mashed Cauliflower
    ½ cup Coconut Oil
    ½ cup Thai Kitchen Coconut Milk Lite
    2 cup Triple Berry Blend
    1 ½ cup Water

INSTRUCTIONS:

In a saucepan, bring fruit and water to boil. Mash the fruit and allow water to boil off (about 20 minutes). In a food processor, combine and mix ingredients for the crust. Spoon the mixture evenly into a cup cake tin and compress with a measuring cup. Remove filling nuts from water. Combine filling ingredients in a processor and blend smooth. Spoon evenly onto crusts. Spoon the fruit mixture on top and using a knife or the spoon swirl the mix. Place the whole thing in the freezer overnight. Use a fork to carefully remove them once frozen.

VARIATIONS/SUGGESTIONS:

- If storing them in the freezer, remove a few hours prior to serving.

BASIC NUTRITION AND KEY VITAMINS/MINERALS PER SERVING							
Calories	Carbs (g)	Net Carbs (g)	Sugar (g)	Protein (g)	Fiber (g)	Fat (g)	Vitamins/Mineral
339	32	25	19	6	7	24	C, E, Potassium

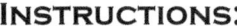

Index